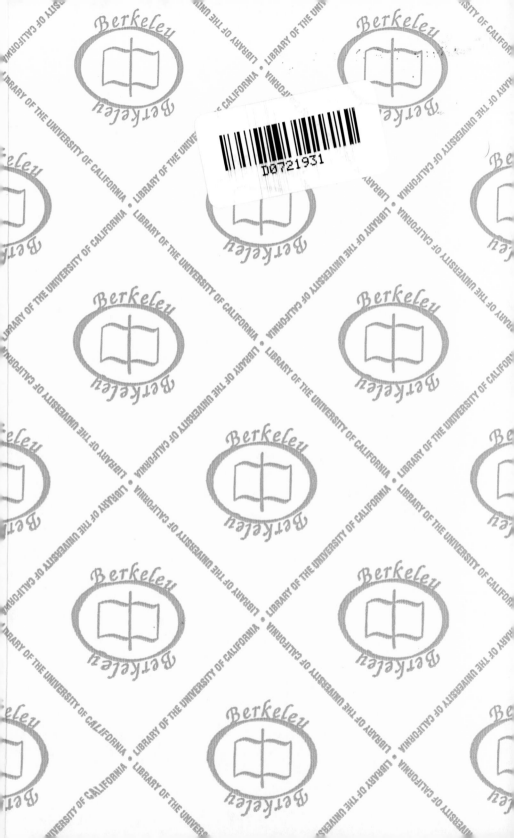

SELF-ESTEEM

AND ADJUSTING
WITH BLINDNESS

SELF-ESTEEM AND ADJUSTING WITH BLINDNESS

The Process of Responding to Life's Demands

By

DEAN W. TUTTLE, Ph.D.

Professor of Special Education
University of Northern Colorado
Greeley, Colorado

With a Foreword by

Gil L. Johnson, M.A.

Director of Client Services
San Francisco Lighthouse for the Blind
San Francisco, California

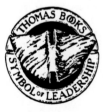

C H A R L E S C T H O M A S • P U B L I S H E R
Springfield • Illinois • U.S.A.

Published and Distributed Throughout the World by
CHARLES C THOMAS • PUBLISHER
2600 South First Street
Springfield, Illinois 62717

© *1984 by* CHARLES C THOMAS • PUBLISHER
ISBN 0-398-04887-8
Library of Congress Catalog Card Number: 83-5037

With THOMAS BOOKS *careful attention is given to all details of
manufacturing and design. It is the Publisher's desire to present books
that are satisfactory as to their physical qualities and artistic possibilities
and appropriate for their particular use.* THOMAS BOOKS *will be true to
those laws of quality that assure a good name and good will.*

Library of Congress Cataloging in Publication Data

Tuttle, Dean W.
  Self-esteem and adjusting with blindness.

  Bibliography: p.
  Includes index.
  1. Blindness—Psychological aspects. 2. Self-respect. 3. Blind—Reha-
bilitation. I. Title. [DNLM: 1. Blindness. 2. Self concept. 3. Adaptation,
Psychological. WW 276 T967s]
HV1593.T87 1984   362.4'12'019   83-5037
ISBN 0-398-04887-8

Printed in the United States of America
PS-R-13

CREDITS FOR QUOTED MATERIAL

v

To Naomi
and
To Ray, Wes, and Rod

FOREWORD

Self-Esteem and Adjusting with Blindness is a book that makes a significant contribution to the understanding of blindness. The way in which a person who is blind feels about himself, self-esteem, is greatly influenced by the attitudes about blindness held by himself and by those important in his life, his adaptability, and the realities with which he must cope. The ways in which these factors affect the self-concept and self-esteem of blind persons are discussed in depth and illustrated with biographical and autobiographical statements from the writings of more than fifty blind persons. When it was begun, the book was primarily intended for use as a textbook for graduate university students. While satisfying this need, the book will be valuable to a much wider audience. It presents a clear and concise introduction for those with experience in other professions who are entering the field of work with the blind. In addition, the book offers an excellent review and update for experienced practitioners and administrators in the field of blindness. The principles set forth are applicable to education, social work, vocational counseling, rehabilitation teaching, recreation therapy, ophthalmology, optometry, and other disciplines.

Too frequently a blind student does not acquire the skills that a teacher "knows" the student could learn or a client of rehabilitation does not achieve the goal of becoming employed. All too often, in such cases, insufficient attention has been given to the level of self-confidence or self-esteem that the student or rehabilitation client has. Some blind persons (consumers) maintain that all that a blind person needs to succeed is an equal opportunity to learn or to obtain a job. It is true that for many the elimination of prejudicial attitudes and equalization of opportunity is all that is needed to enable a blind individual to achieve his potential. Many others need something more. They often need guidance and support to go through the stages of adjusting to blindness and to develop the prerequisite feelings of self-worth or self-esteem before they can achieve their goals. The book describes the steps in this process and discusses the important role of the professional. *Self-Esteem and Adjusting with Blindness* represents a major step in the drawing together of the discipline of psychology and sociology into the education and rehabilitation of blind children and adults.

Gil L. Johnson, M.A.

PREFACE

In the past, a great deal has been written about blind persons, their early development, educational needs, employment opportunities, and their ability in general to meet life's demands in a sighted society. Biographies and autobiographies of blind persons account for more than a hundred books within the available array of literature. Some of this literature is objective and factual while some is subjective and emotional; some is research-based, some opinion-based; some is fragmented, lacking a basic construct that permits one to understand and interrelate the many bits and parts of the complex process, some provides a more global and cohesive theoretical structure.

Self-Esteem and Adjusting with Blindness is an attempt to analyze blindness within the context of two overlapping theoretical constructs: the development of self-esteem and the adjusting process to social and/or physical trauma. The book is divided into four sections. The first provides a brief overview of blindness, an essential background for subsequent discussions. Section II proposes a general theoretical model for the development of self-esteem common to all persons and attempts to analyze the impact that blindness imposes upon this model. Section III analyzes the process of coping with social and physical traumas or crises, and the way in which self-esteem is affected by the adjusting process. Section IV is addressed to the professional and/or lay person who has frequent contact with the blind child or adult. It provides some hints and suggestions for creating a climate for the optimum development of a strong and positive sense of self-esteem in the blind individual.

The title *Self-Esteem and Adjusting with Blindness* may be misleading. A better title would be "A Study of the Relationship Between a Person's Self-Esteem and the Process of Adjusting to Life's Demands with the Personal Attribute of Blindness," but it is obviously too long. One does not adjust *to* blindness as though blindness were some external circumstance, as when one adjusts to a new job or a new home. Blindness is only one of many personal attributes that make up the total person, and it is the total person who is engaged in meeting life's demands.

Although the author is himself blind, he does not claim any special insights as a result of losing his vision during adolescence and young adulthood. Rather, the book grows out of twenty years of working as a professional in the education and rehabilitation of blind children and young adults.

The author is indebted to the many capable blind persons who wrote of their own personal experiences or who shared for others to write. Although most of the biographies and autobiographies are written in retrospect, and thus subject to filtered interpretations of remembered experiences, the illustrations chosen represent a larger collection of events common to many. The biographical excerpts are not offered to prove a theoretical model but serve only to illustrate it. A list of the biographies and autobiographies reviewed for this book can be found in the bibliography.

D.W.T

ACKNOWLEDGMENTS

Many have contributed to the development of this book, both directly and indirectly. My parents, Glen and Jeannette Tuttle, have been a constant source of support and encouragement. My mentor through graduate school in special education, Georgie Lee Abel, has contributed to the basic philosophy and attitudes toward visual impairments reflected in the book.

My deep appreciation is extended to Gil Johnson who agreed to review the manuscript to offer suggestions from the rehabilitation perspective. Gil's sensitivity and insights regarding the issues under consideration have earned him national respect.

Other professional colleagues have contributed in many different ways. I am indebted

to Gid and Martha Jones of Florida State University for help in the book's early development;

to my fellow faculty in Special Education at the University of Northern Colorado for their advice and counsel, and especially to Dave Kappan for his critique of the orientation and mobility sections;

to Jennifer Hill, an experienced teacher of visually impaired children, for her review and helpful comments;

to Carol Ann Moore, a journalist and colleague in the reading department, for her editorial assistance;

and to Buck Schrotberger, Colorado consultant for the visually impaired, for his analysis of significant others' reactions to trauma.

Finally, the book would not have been possible without the persistent and untiring efforts of my wife. The extensive library research, the dictation taken from my braille copy, the editorial assistance during the many revisions and the typing of the final manuscript are a credit to her versatile abilities. Her background in the nursing profession, her experience with many disabled persons, and her observations of others' reactions to the disabled have provided valuable insights into the subtle and sensitive topics that are handled in the book.

D.W.T.

CONTENTS

Page

Forward xi

Preface xiii

Section I—A DEFINITION OF BLINDNESS

Chapter

1 AN OVERVIEW OF BLINDNESS 5

Blindness and Self-esteem 5

Historical Perspective 8

Terminology 12

Extreme Variability 14

Prevalence and Incidence 16

Summary 17

2 THE IMPACT OF BLINDNESS 18

Implications for Personal and Home Management .. 21

Implications for Travel 22

Implications for Reading and Writing 29

Vocational Implications 32

Implications for Recreation 35

Summary 37

3 PSYCHOSOCIAL IMPLICATIONS OF
BLINDNESS 38

Sociological Implications 38

Psychological Implications........................ 49
Summary... 57

Section II—THE DEVELOPMENT OF SELF-ESTEEM

4   SOURCES OF SELF-ESTEEM, EXTERNALLY
     ORIENTED...................................... 61
     Self, Self-concept, and Self-esteem 62
     Self-esteem and Reflections 66
     Self-esteem and Relationships..................... 82
     Self-esteem and Self-appraisal.................... 88
     Summary... 90
5   SOURCES OF SELF-ESTEEM, INTERNALLY
     ORIENTED 91
     VI's Aspirations and SO's Expectations........... 94
     VI's Performance and Observed Performance 98
     Self-evaluation and Evaluation by Others 101
     Responses to Evaluations: Success or Failure...... 107
     Value Priorities 111
     Basic Drives and Developmental Needs 115
     Summary.. 118
6   SELF-ESTEEM AND THE RESOLUTION
     OF DISCREPANCIES......................... 121
     Sources of Discrepancies and Anxieties 123
     Reactions to Discrepancies 126
     The Resolution of Discrepancies.................. 128
     Defense Mechanisms 136
     Characteristics of High and Low Self-esteem 137
     Summary.. 142

Section III—ADJUSTING WITH BLINDNESS

7   THE ADJUSTING PROCESS 145
     The Meaning of Adjustment 146
     Qualitative Adjustment 149
     Models of Adjusting with Blindness.............. 151
     Summary.. 157

Contents   xix

8   SEQUENTIAL MODEL OF ADJUSTING
     WITH BLINDNESS 159
     Phase One: Trauma, Physical or Social 160
     Phase Two: Shock and Denial.................... 170
     Phase Three: Mourning and Withdrawal 175
     Phase Four: Succumbing and Depression 181
     Phase Five: Reassessment and Reaffirmation 193
     Phase Six: Coping and Mobilization.............. 205
     Phase Seven: Self-acceptance and Self-esteem 223
     Summary....................................... 236
9   FACTORS INFLUENCING THE ADJUSTING
     PROCESS 239
     Factors Internal to the Individual 239
     Factors External to the Individual 253
     Degree of Independence and Level of Self-esteem .. 262
     Summary....................................... 275

        Section IV—FOSTERING SELF-ESTEEM

10   GUIDELINES AND SUGGESTED ACTIVITIES . 279
     Guidelines for Working with Blind Persons 280
     Attitudes and Behaviors that Foster Affective
     Growth 284
     Activities to Stimulate Affective Growth 287
Bibliography 297
Index... 311

SELF-ESTEEM
AND ADJUSTING
WITH BLINDNESS

Section I
A DEFINITION
OF BLINDNESS

Chapter 1

AN OVERVIEW OF BLINDNESS

T he experience of blindness is both a physical and a psychosocial phenomenon. The medical component provides data regarding etiology, diagnosis, prescription, and prognosis. However, it is more important that the experience of blindness be described in terms of the inter-action among three elements: the needs and desires of an individual with little or no vision; the physical and social environment of an individual; and the common conception of blindness. In order to understand better the interactive process, one must first come to grips with the concept and dynamics of blindness.

BLINDNESS AND SELF-ESTEEM

The title, *Self-Esteem and Adjusting with Blindness*, may erroneously suggest to some readers that self-esteem is a problem unique to blind persons. Of course, nothing could be further from the truth. The needs for food and shelter, for love and belonging, for responsibility and productivity, for self-acceptance and self-esteem are universal regardless of whether the individual is blind or sighted. The factors that contribute to anyone's self-esteem are the same ones that contribute to a blind person's self-esteem. The way one feels about himself influences the way he is able to perform, and his performance, in turn, affects the way he feels about himself and the way others perceive him. The way others perceive him impacts on the way he feels about himself and

5

thus, the way he is able to perform. Self-esteem and competence are the keys to successfully meeting life's demands. However, blindness contributes some added dynamics deserving special attention.

> The real pain I was beginning to feel was not physical, it was spiritual. It was a loss of self-esteem. That thing I call the elephant was really a big creature with a shriveled self-image. He did not think well of himself. He felt guilty. He felt inadequate. He felt unable to cope. Those are surefire self-esteem problems. (Kemper, 1977, p. 67)

Kemper, a recently blinded adult, described how his self-esteem was affected by his blindness. The term *self-esteem* refers to a person's sense of value and worth, his sense of competence and adequacy, his sense of self-satisfaction. For most people, the dominant role that vision plays in the performance of daily tasks is taken for granted. When sight is lost, the person feels particularly helpless and dependent until he can acquire appropriate adaptive behaviors and coping skills. At the same time, the minimal expectations and negative attitudes experienced by the blind person contribute to lowered self-esteem. Thus, the dynamic forces that operate upon a newly blinded person make his sense of worth and competence especially vulnerable.

The development of self-esteem among those born blind is also precarious. All children growing up, especially through their teen years, wrestle with the fundamental questions: "Who am I?", "Am I lovable?", "What is the meaning of life?", "Where do I belong?", "Can I handle it?" The blind child who experiences devaluating and derogatory reactions or reflections within his social environment finds it more difficult to obtain satisfactory answers to these basic issues of life. When any child is made to feel strange, different, unwanted, incapable, or inadequate, his self-esteem is jeopardized.

> From the other side of the road I heard the voices of little boys and the sound of something else—a ball bouncing against a wall or wooden gate. I called out, "Hello! Can I play with you? Can I come and play?"
> The ball stopped bouncing and there was silence. Then one of the

boys answered, "No, you can't. You couldn't play if you tried. Cross-Eyes!"

As I turned and felt my way back to the house, I heard the ball start bouncing again. (Hocken, 1977, pp. 1-2)

When Hocken sensed that she was unwanted and that she was different in some way from the rest of the children, her self-esteem was affected, either consciously or unconsciously. Childhood experiences that help to formulate a person's self-esteem can have long-lasting influence. Many years later Hocken was still struggling with her sense of value and worth.

But the doubts remained. Don could see. I was blind. Therefore he could not possibly be in love with me. The logic seemed inescapable. At the same time I was certain, yet skeptical, of my own love for him. Love was something I had read about in braille paperbacks, and invariably concerned sighted people. How could it happen to me? (Hocken, 1977, p. 95)

Self-esteem does not need to be any more of a problem for a blind person than for anyone else in society. Many who have struggled with basic self-esteem issues of life have resolved them satisfactorily.

We learn to get the most out of what we have and to work around what we lack. Actually we're like everybody else in that respect. Most of us manage to climb up to some kind of plateau on which we find some degree of self-satisfaction and security. Some of us are satisfied to stay there, feeling lucky to have gotten anywhere at all. Others want to climb higher. As you have seen, the problems arise when we are prevented from making the most of our lives. (Sperber, 1976, p. 213)

The intent of this book is to identify the factors that contribute to high self-esteem, in order to capitalize on them, and to analyze the factors that contribute to low self-esteem, in order to minimize their effects. When one considers that a source of self-esteem is to be found in reflections (see Chapter 4), the prevailing attitudes and feelings about blindness held by others become critical. If self-esteem is measured in terms of one's feeling of competence or adequacy (see Chapter 5), blind children and adults are frequently made to feel anything but competent or adequate. The adjusting process (see Chapter 8) describes a person's reaction to a severe trauma whether that trauma is the initial onset of blindness or a confrontation with derogatory and devaluating attitudes about blindness. While the recently blinded is adjusting to a new condition, the child born blind is adjusting to initial and subsequent confrontations with the social stigma of blindness. Some of the phases of adjusting with blindness, such as mourning or succumbing, may involve withdrawal or depression—potential contributors to lowered self-esteem.

Adjusting with blindness can be viewed as a process of adjusting to life's demands with the added stress of blindness for both the child born blind and the person blinded later. It is a continual life-long process in which parents, teachers, rehabilitation workers, medical personnel, and others all contribute to the individual's search for self-acceptance and self-esteem. The role of the professional in the adjusting process and specific suggestions for fostering self-acceptance and self-esteem are presented in this book, to assist in the educational and rehabilitation effort. A review of the historical perspectives regarding the status and treatment of blind people provides some necessary insights into the social dynamics that impinge upon the individual blind person both in the past and in the present.

HISTORICAL PERSPECTIVE

Although blind persons do not yet enjoy the same full and equal status accorded most other members of society, there have been remarkable changes, particularly in the past two centuries. In the book *The Changing Status of the Blind*, Lowenfeld (1975) identified four phases in society's treatment of blind persons: separation, ward status, self-emancipation, and integration. The subsequent discussion follows the same general format; however the ward status has been renamed "protection," and the last phase has been divided into two separate topics, education and assimilation.

Separation

There was a time in antiquity when most blind persons were ostracized or annihilated from society. The prevailing unchallenged assumption that blind persons could not contribute to the welfare of the community survival needs mandated this harsh treatment. "The blind" were not seen as people but as objects that were threatening to society; thus society was able to rationalize its cruel behavior.

Protection

During the Judiac and early Christian periods, pity and compassion for the blind began to emerge as dominant patterns. Recognition of the blind as members of the human race brought with it the responsibility to care for one's brother. This care and concern found expression in the establishment of asylums or sheltered environments where the basic needs for food, clothing, and housing were met. Although protection would be preferred to annihilation, it represented another form of annihilation—that of the soul. Care and nurture of the body are not the same as care and nurture of the personality. Although now recognized as members of society, blind persons were still not perceived as capable of contributing to the welfare of society. The dignity and worth of the blind person remained in doubt and the natural consequence was lowered self-esteem of the individual.

Self-Emancipation

During the seventeenth and eighteenth centuries, there were several blind persons who, through their own efforts, rose to prominence despite the prevailing attitudes. A musician, Friedrich Ludwig Dulon; a lawyer, Nicholas Bacon; a mathematician, John Gough; a philosopher, Huldreich Schonberger; and an engineer, John Metcalf, among others proved that blind persons could contribute to the welfare of their communities (Lowenfeld, 1975). Although these individuals were exceptions, they proved that blind persons were capable of learning.

Education

Since it was demonstrated that blind persons were capable of being educated, the next logical step was to establish training facilities for the blind. The schools that were established during the nineteenth century were primarily residential—where blind children lived away from home and attended classes segregated from their sighted peers. With the development of specialized reading and writing systems and other adaptive aids, blind children demonstrated their capability of learning not only academic subjects but also vocational skills.

However, there was still no open acceptance of blind persons within society at large. Blind persons were allowed to be productive as long as they were productive in their place. For many this meant menial, repetitive jobs such as broom-making or chair-caning within a sheltered workshop environment. The feelings of being worthy, of being valuable to the community were, by and large, still unrealized by most blind persons, and society did not attempt to foster the healthy attitudes taken for granted by the sighted population.

> My increasing interest in teaching and betterment of the blind impelled me to concentrate in sociology. Prior to state and federally sponsored welfare programs in the mid-thirties, it was not uncommon for some blind to go "on the stem" as it was called. They sold pencils or shoe strings, or sang or played instruments on street corners for whatever the sympathetic public might contribute. When a capable, close friend did this to eke out an existence for himself, his wife, and child, I was determined to do something about such an unsatisfactory means of making a living. It made the blind an object of pity while it robbed the seeing of a constructive attitude toward helping blind people achieve gainful employment and equality of opportunity. (Fries, 1980, p. 210)

Assimilation

The failure of the blind to be assimilated into society was

perhaps because the blind had not learned to compete with the sighted at school. At the same time, sighted people had had no opportunity to experience the full potential of blind individuals. The education of blind children in the twentieth century began focusing on integrating blind children with sighted children in the public schools. Blind children became members of the regular classroom, taught with their sighted peers, yet receiving specialized instruction as needed from a teacher trained to work with the blind. Approximately 75 percent of the blind children in the United States are currently educated in the public schools. Many visually handicapped children have found the experience of attending classes with sighted peers to be personally, socially, and academically enriching and satisfying. However, physical integration does not necessarily result in social integration. The physical presence of a blind child in the classroom with his sighted peers does not guarantee his acceptance by them.

> I once knew a little boy who spent a million recess periods standing right in the middle of a windswept playground just praying that someone—anyone—would notice him and knowing all the time that nobody would.
> I once knew a child who sent Valentine cards to every person in the whole class and received not a single one in return.
> I once knew an adolescent who always sat at an empty table in a junior high school cafeteria pretending that he wasn't even aware that he was sitting next to emptiness.
> I once knew a teen-ager who spent days waiting for the telephone to ring, but it never did, and who spent Saturday nights alone with his radio pretending he was listening to it.
> I once knew a man who was afraid that because he happened not to see, he would be consigned to an eternity of loneliness where there would be nobody who would want to marry him. (Krents, 1972, p. 11)

Furthermore, integration in the schools does not necessarily result in assimilation into adult society. In spite of the education and rehabilitation efforts of the twentieth century, full assimilation into society is far from being achieved (Lowenfeld, 1975). When a blind person's basic need to belong to the world around him remains unfulfilled, his self-esteem suffers.

I was experiencing what most blind people experience sooner or later. They want—but "want" isn't strong enough; "need" is a better word—they need to belong to the world around them. All of us, while apparently separate and distinct individuals, are but the molecules of which the body of humanity is composed, and each of us feels a compulsion to function as a part of the whole. Consciously or subconsciously we long to be useful and accepted, regarded with favor. Loss of sight does not change this, I discovered; I needed to find a way to belong.

What could I do? (Carver, 1961, p. 178)

The struggle continues. The level of self-esteem of blind persons is a function of the degree of assimilation they experience in society, a measure of the dignity and worth of the individual (Resnick, 1981). This is not to imply that everyone in modern society shares the attitude that would foster the assimilation of all blind persons. There are some who would prefer to separate, to protect, and to educate the blind without acknowledging the fundamental right of every blind person to be a fully participating member of society. However, with increased assimilation, it is hoped that there will be increased acceptance.

TERMINOLOGY

Vision can be conceptualized as ranging on a continuum from normal vision (NV) to totally blind (TB). Normal vision has a Snellen measured acuity of 20/20 and a visual field that subtends an arc of 160 to 180 degrees. The literature refers to partially seeing (PS) persons as those individuals whose visual acuity with best correction in the better eye ranges between 20/70 and 20/200. The person with a visual acuity of 20/70 must approach an object to within 20 feet to see it as clearly as another person with normal vision could see it at 70 feet.

The 1935 Social Security Act established the definition of "legally blind" (LB) in the United States, a definition still commonly held today. It has two parts, either of which is sufficient by itself to qualify a person as being legally blind: (1) a Snellen visual acuity of 20/200 or less in the better eye with best correction or (2) restriction in the field of vision such that the widest diameter of the visual field subtends an arc no greater than 20 degrees. Barraga (1976) indicated that 75-80 percent of the legally blind population have sufficient residual vision to be able to use it as a primary learning channel. These individuals are "low vision" persons. Figure 1 summarizes the relationship among the commonly used terms.

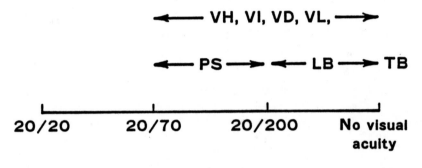

Figure 1. Terminology

There are four terms used more or less synonymously that refer to individuals with a visual loss requiring modification of life-style: visually impaired (VI), visually handicapped (VH), visually disabled (VD), and visually limited (VL). Nevertheless, some subtle differences exist. Wright (1960) differentiated between "handicap" and "disability" by stating that a handicap was an obstacle to the attainment of a desired goal whereas a disability referred only to the physiological, medically measurable loss of vision.

This connotation of the word handicap is still in common usage. Blindness may or may not be a handicap. If a blind person's goal were to be a jet pilot, then blindness would be a handicap. A parent who is ashamed of blindness may require that his blind child behave in every way as though he could see, an unrealistic goal, and thus a handicap for both parent and child. On the other hand, for the blind person who delivers a speech or engages in recreational swimming, blindness should impose no handicap.

The determination of blindness as an obstacle can either

be self-imposed or imposed by others. A newly blind person may give up his teaching position because he mistakenly believes blind people are incapable of being successful teachers. On the other hand, a blind person's desire to practice law might be thwarted because a law firm discriminated against blind persons.

> I quickly discovered that finding employment with a law firm was going to be about as easy as regaining my vision. . . .
> There would be about ten lawyers gathered in a huge conference room, filled with acrid cigar smoke. The reaction would always be the same—irritation verging on hostility that I should even presume to think that a blind person could possibly function as an associate in their firm.
> "Mr. Krents, I think it only fair to begin this interview by stating that as far as we are concerned, there is not only no legal position available here for you, but it is our belief that there is no place in the legal profession where a blind person could operate successfully." I ran into this attitude on other occasions. (Krents, 1972, p. 277)

Thus blindness can be a handicap in one of two ways: (1) unrealistic goals in view of the realistic impact of blindness and (2) unrealistic restrictions ascribed to blindness. Section II will discuss the social origins of both problems.

The word *disabled* in more recent years has taken on a different connotation than was used by Wright (1960). A disabled car is unable to move under its own power even though it may only be the carburetor that is malfunctioning. The current implication of the word disabled seems to include total incapacity (Kirtley, 1975). For this reason the term "visual disability" may carry with it some connotations that tend to decrease self-esteem.

Since blindness in and of itself does not incapacitate the person, there was a need for another term to refer to the physiological medically measurable loss of vision. Visually impaired or visually limited served this purpose. However, given time, these two terms may take on new meanings.

EXTREME VARIABILITY

The terminology just discussed is insufficient to capture the extreme variability among visually impaired persons.

Some individuals are blind from birth, congenitally blind, such as those with congenital cataracts. Others lose their vision later, adventitiously blinded, as with macular degeneration. Some causes affect just the vision (e.g. detached retina), while others have a systemic origin (e.g. diabetes). In certain instances blindness is sudden and traumatic although not necessarily total (e.g. car accident), and in others, the loss is gradual over months, years, or even a lifetime (e.g. retinitis pigmentosa).

> My eyesight was still not an incapacitating problem.... During the day, I would make dates to dance with various lady guests, but come night and I couldn't see well enough to walk, let alone dance. Those who came to the dance regularly knew I had a problem and understood my strange predicament. They tried to be helpful as best they could. (Sperber, 1976, p. 29)

Some visual impairments are obvious to an observer, others are not. For example, someone with tunnel vision may be legally blind but have a central visual acuity of 20/20, enabling him to read normal print at normal distances, but he encounters difficulties travelling without a white cane. Another legally blind person may have sufficient residual vision to travel without a cane but be unable to read regular print. Certain conditions require higher levels of illumination for optimum visibility while others need lower levels of illumination. Some visually limited persons can be helped in performing visual tasks by the use of magnifiers or electronic enlargers while others cannot. For some, the visual loss is stable or becomes stabilized through medical intervention while the vision of others fluctuates from day to day or from setting to setting.

> My occasional ability to decipher detail—newly applied mascara, a wrinkle, the sparkle of an earring—depends on the momentary coming together of several ideal conditions: the intensity of light, the relationship of figure to ground, my distance and angle of sight. These momentary flashes of accurate vision combine incongruously with my inability to cross a street safely or avoid colliding with a tree on a simple country walk. The unevenness of sight confuses me and those close to me: at times I can perceive and report minutiae, at other times I see nothing. (Potok, 1980, p. 42)

This variability is compounded by the degree to which one

has learned how to use his residual vision effectively. Visual efficiency is to be distinguished from visual acuity (Barraga, 1980). Two visually impaired children with identical visual acuity may respond quite differently to their visual surroundings. One who has not learned or is unwilling to use the residual vision may respond minimally if at all to the visual world around him. The other may rely exclusively on the visual stimuli.

The extreme variability in the extent and manner of visual loss is little understood by the general public and often becomes a basis for misunderstanding. A casual observer may be perplexed upon seeing a person with low vision walking confidently to a bus stop yet having to ask the driver for the number of the bus, or upon seeing a blind person with excellent mobility skills able to travel independently in a familiar setting and yet requiring assistance in another setting, or upon waving to a low vision person and receiving no response. This misunderstanding can lead to confused or disturbed interpersonal relationships (see Chapter 4). It can also result in an identity problem for the visually impaired person (see Chapter 8).

> In school, I gradually came to realize that the other boys and girls had an easier time of things. I knew that I had to put my face right up to a book to learn to read, but I could see the shape of Trudy, who sat next to me, holding her book away from her. Not only that, she giggled and asked, "What are you smelling your book for, Sheila?"...
>
> So I held the book away, but the print immediately blurred. I brought it back to my face again and discovered reassuringly, that the Cat remained firmly on the Mat. "I'm not silly" I insisted. (Hocken, 1977, p. 6)

PREVALENCE AND INCIDENCE

There are two commonly accepted statistical guidelines for the prevalence of blind persons in the United States: (1) Within the school age population there is one legally blind child for every 1,000 school children (0.1%) (Gearheart, 1980); (2) Within the general population there are two legally blind persons for every 1,000 (0.2%) (National Society to Prevent Blindness, 1980). As age increases, the incidence rate of newly blinded persons increases, as illustrated in Figure 2. Approximately 50 percent of all blind people are over the age of sixty-five, and 65 percent of all blind people are over fifty years of age (National Society to Prevent Blindness, 1980; Kirchner and Peterson, 1981).

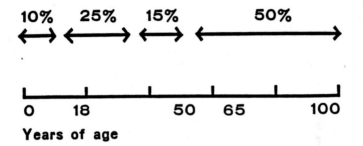

Figure 2. Age Distribution of the Legally Blind in the United States

The low incidence and prevalence figures introduce other problems. Blind children have little chance to learn about the realistic impact of blindness and how best to cope with it from other blind children in their home community (see Chapter 9). Rather, they are forced to use the trial-and-error discovery process or rely on the possibly unrealistic perceptions of the sighted persons around them. The sighted, too, it must be recognized, have little opportunity to interact with a wide variety of visually impaired persons in their community. Consequently, the perceptions of sighted persons about blindness are generally left to the imagination, an unreliable source of realistic data.

SUMMARY

From the historical perspective, the climate of the development of feelings of self-worth among persons who are blind has improved but is far from optimal. Unrealistic perceptions of blindness and the extreme variability of the nature of visual losses among visually impaired persons are sources of confusion. Blind persons represent a small number in any community, thus giving them a feeling of uniqueness and resulting in a sense of being different. Feelings of differentness often precipitate problems with self-esteem.

Chapter 2

THE IMPACT OF BLINDNESS

The impact of blindness must first be understood from the perspective of the required adaptations in lifestyle that result directly from the physiological loss of vision in and of itself, whether this loss be partial or total. Then the impact must be understood within the context of society's prevailing attitude. The self-concept and self-esteem of a person who is visually impaired emerge from his interaction with the physical and social environment.

Kirtley (1975) described two polarized views of the impact of blindness, with many blind people holding positions somewhere between these two extremes.

On the one hand, there are those who see blindness as a virtual disaster. This group stresses the physical, psychological, and social limitations associated with blindness and considers it a tragic fate that can never be substantially overcome without superior ability and/or unusually favorable environmental circumstances. The blind person is seen as essentially different from the seeing individual.... At the opposite pole, there are others who assess blindness as nothing more than a physical nuisance or practical inconvenience. They contend that the problems traditionally linked to blindness are almost totally the product of social prejudice and discrimination, that blindness, in itself, is at most only a minor handicap. Indeed the proponents of this view resent the very use of such words as handicap, disability and impairment in connection with blindness.... The first view tends to be pessimistic and defeatist, fostering in those blind who accept it an unproductive orientation toward passivity, gloomy resignation, and childlike dependency on the seeing. On the other hand, the second position involves an unrealistic degree of optimism,

for certain obvious handicapping effects of blindness are simply
denied or ignored. (pp. 137-138)

It is difficult to define the nature of the impact, the extent
of the impact, and the source of the impact, whether the
more realistic direct effects of impaired vision or the more
unrealistic socially determined consequences. No one will
disagree that blindness impinges upon or alters the life-
style of an individual in meeting the practical day-to-day
demands of living. The needs of visually impaired persons
are the same needs shared by all persons, and many of these
are satisfied in the very same way. Some needs, however,
the visually impaired meet by employing techniques and
methods different from those of their sighted peers. It is this
differentness that tends to be disturbing to one's self-
esteem. The fact that a blind child or adult accomplishes
certain tasks in a manner different from the sighted should
not be reflected in judgments of one's value and competence.

A blind person's self-esteem is also affected by the
recognition that he is not totally self-sufficient, that he is
dependent on the sighted to meet some of his needs even
with the best adaptive behaviors and coping skills. The
dependency needs of the blind are more visible or more
obvious than the dependency needs of the sighted, and as a
result, most members of society tend to share the opinion
that the visually impaired are more dependent and thus less
worthy. The sighted find it easy to forget that interdependence is healthy and normal (see Chapter 9). There is
abundant evidence to support the conviction that visually
impaired children and adults can be capable, contributing
members of their society. With the proper conditions, a blind
child can develop into an independent, responsible, freely
functioning individual (Norris et al., 1957). The fact that
blindness in and of itself does not impede mental growth is
amply proven by the successes of many prominent blind
persons throughout history (Kirtley, 1975).

Yet, there are some potential problem areas enroute
toward achieving competency. Lowenfeld (1963) described
three basic limitations that blindness imposes on the

individual: (1) the limitation in the range and variety of experiences; (2) the limitation in the ability to get about; and (3) the limitation in the control of the environment and the self in relation to it" (p. 90). These "basic limitations" impact broadly upon a person's life and will be discussed in the following areas: (1) implications for personal and home management, (2) implications for travel, (3) implications for reading and writing, (4) vocational implications, and (5) recreational implications.

A person with impaired vision, either partial or total, requires accommodation to some extent in each of the above areas. As a general rule, the greater the visual loss, the more extensive and divergent are the coping techniques required for successful accommodation. Thus, the totally blind may find it more difficult to acquire the necessary adaptive skills (such as use of braille for reading and writing and the white cane for travel) while the techniques such as use of felt tip pen and hand magnifier employed by low vision persons are less difficult to acquire and more similar to the techniques used by the general public. However, the low vision person frequently finds himself having more difficulty with the psychosocial adjusting process (to be discussed later). Since the low vision person may appear as though he were normally sighted, his behavior is more frequently misunderstood. Such misunderstanding produces ambiguities, embarrassments, and conflicts that lead to personal traumas. Thus, from a psychosocial perspective, the low vision person tends to find the adjusting process toward self-acceptance and self-esteem more difficult.

> One day as I worked in the store I had a chat with Norvall Freese who sold band instruments and sheet music. He was working his way through college, too, so I suggested that he could read to me for pay. He looked up from his stooped position and replied, "I don't have time to do that but why don't you do your own reading?"
> "Why Norvall, I can't see to read. All I can read is Braille!"
> As if in amazement, he said, "I'll be damned! That's why you high-hatted me the other day."
> "What do you mean?"
> "I waved to you on the street and you didn't even smile at me. From

that I figured you could go your way and I would go mine." (Fries, 1980, pp. 180-181)

IMPLICATIONS FOR PERSONAL AND HOME MANAGEMENT

Developing adequate competence and independence in personal and home management skills is a universal concern for both congenitally and adventitiously blind persons. For the congenitally blind, the responsibility for guiding these learning experiences rests with their parents and, later, their teachers (Suterko, 1973). The adventitiously blind adult learns these skills by receiving instructions either at an orientation center for the blind or from a rehabilitation teacher in his own home.

These techniques of daily living cover a variety of topics including personal care and grooming, dressing, eating, care of clothing, house cleaning, cooking, sewing, home repairs, etc. To the sighted, these skills may appear to be superficial and elementary. To the visually impaired who are limited in their ability to learn by visual observation and imitation, these skills are obstacles to independence unless specifically taught and mastered (Tuttle, 1981a).

For the blind child, these skills must be mastered without the benefit of observation and imitation. For the newly blinded adult it means learning to do in a new and initially strange manner some old familiar routine tasks such as folding paper money by denominations, pinning pairs of socks together, color coding clothes, pouring liquids by touch, vacuuming in a grid pattern, using oven mitts.

From what I have said, I do not want to give the impression that my life had become cumbersome. It simply meant that I had to find new ways of doing things, and then train myself to get used to them. I was sure that if I exercised enough energy, patience and (I hope) intelligence, I would begin to live almost as naturally as I did before...

I would work out all sorts of devices to get along, and some of them would be unorthodox. I had always had to approach my problems in a different way from people who had good vision, and that had never prevented me from getting along as well as most and having a good time doing it. (Dahl, 1962, pp. 69, 10)

For the blind child as well as for the newly blinded adult, mastery over and responsibility for daily home chores provide a sense of accomplishment and personal satisfaction. Feelings of heightened self-esteem and self-worth emerge from being able to contribute to the welfare of the home and being able to manage other personal needs.

> I did other little odd jobs while I was home. None of them very difficult; but all of them terrifically important to my morale. Each new thing I did gave me new confidence. (Fox, 1946, pp. 157-158)

Until the techniques of daily living become routine—that is, until they can be accomplished without concentrated mental and physical energies—they will require more time and result in greater mental and physical fatigue (Roberts, 1973).

For parents and teachers, there is always the temptation to do the job oneself to save time and avoid stress, thus depriving the child of valuable practice.

> It would seem strange to me if I weren't able to do these things. Perhaps I wouldn't be able to do them if Mother hadn't been so wise, so unselfish, and so foresighted. She dedicated herself to making me as self-reliant and independent as possible. She often said that the hardest thing she ever had to do was NOT to do everything for me after I became blind. (Clifton, 1962, p. 101)

IMPLICATIONS FOR TRAVEL

> I got along the pavement as best I could—and that is another frightening experience difficult to describe to anyone who has not been blind, because though you are surrounded by noise, you have no coherent mental picture of what is around you. Sometimes I could tell by the particular quality of the sounds of traffic and footsteps that I was near buildings or passing an open space. But I had absolutely no idea what the road might be like and still less what might be on the other side of it. Were there children playing, people gossiping, women buying bread or potatoes? What did they look like? Who were they? I could not imagine any of it. I walked along in an enclosed gray little world, a two-foot-square box of sounds around me. (Hocken, 1977, p. 25)

One of the most significant and immediate consequences of blindness has to do with one's ability to travel through one's physical and social environment, to anticipate and, thus, to exercise some control over potentially hazardous situations in that environment. The development of these skills is accomplished through instruction in orientation and mobility. Orientation is the ability to create and maintain a mental map of one's environment and the relationship of oneself to that environment. Mobility, on the other hand, is the ability to travel safely and efficiently through that environment.

The visually impaired person—like the sighted person— learns about his environment by interacting with it beginning in infancy and continuing throughout life. It requires movement, exploration, and curiosity utilizing all residual senses and integrating the sensations into a conceptual whole. Barraga (1976) has proposed that "for children who are blind or have low vision, movement may be the most accurate replacement for vision in clarifying information about the world" (p. 25).

With adequate training, pedestrian travel is able to be mastered. There are four primary modes of mobility, each with specific advantages and disadvantages (Kappan, 1981).

Sighted Guide

Some blind persons on occasion choose to walk with a sighted companion. By lightly grasping the companion's arm above the elbow, the blind person thereby places himself a half step behind. If the body movement of the companion is insufficient to indicate step-ups, step-downs, changes of pace or direction, it can be supplemented with verbal communication.

There are some who feel that too much independence is abdicated when using a sighted guide. It conjures up images of extreme dependency when it becomes the sole mode of travel. However, if the blind person is walking with a companion or in a group toward some common destination, a sighted guide is the more relaxed and sociable alternative for all concerned. The degree of dependence is better measured by the degree to which the blind person maintains himself as an active manager or participant of the process rather than simply docile and acquiescent. Even with the best of skills, blind persons sometimes find themselves in awkward situations.

> I have an unfortunate habit, when I am out with somebody and we have to separate for an instant, of grabbing on to the wrong person when I think we are reunited. One night arriving at a dark railway station, I got out of the train just ahead of the friend I was traveling with. Thinking he was still with me, I pushed my arm through another which seemed to be waiting for mine. It belonged to a girl who was startled by the unorthodox approach. Her boyfriend was showing alarming signs of aggression, until he saw my white stick as my companion rescued me from the scene. (Edwards, 1962, pp. 92-93)

The Cane

A majority of blind persons use the white cane as their mode of independent travel. To be a competent cane traveler, one must participate in a rigorous sequence of instruction taught by a trained orientation and mobility specialist. After training, the cane enables one to travel independently as it provides a means for detecting obstacles, step-ups, drop-offs, surface textures, etc., by integrating tactile, kinesthetic, and auditory signals provided by the cane. Mastery of this skill contributes to the individual's sense of competence and self-esteem.

> How much Bob's canes protect him is evident by their beaten-up condition after he has carried them awhile.
> "Every mark on the cane is one not on my shins," he says.
> He has marks on his shins too, and he freely admits that they are there because he hasn't used his cane as effectively as he might. (Moore, 1960, p. 169)

The cane has several disadvantages. It does not detect overhanging obstacles, such as tree branches. The blind person's interaction with the environment is limited to that portion of the environment that the cane contacts, providing fragmented information upon which to develop one's mental map. As a result, when a blind person is in an unfamiliar setting, he must either take time to explore his new surroundings or rely on information provided by someone else.

Dog Guide

There are fewer than ten major dog guide schools in the United States, the oldest of which is Seeing Eye[T.M.], in Morristown, New Jersey. Less than 4 percent of the blind population either desire or qualify for a dog guide (Welsh and Blasch, 1980). The dog is in training for three or more months prior to the four-week training period during which the blind person learns to work with his dog guide. This training is at minimal or no cost to the blind person. A good working relationship with a dog can provide some blind persons with a confidence and freedom of travel that was for that person previously unattainable by any other means. It requires someone who is active, mature, and willing to accept the responsibility for the care and discipline of a dog.

> The despairing emptiness that had entered my heart when blindness had brought me to a complete stop was replaced by a vital interest and a challenge. This new zest for life all stemmed from the moment a warm, wet tongue caressed my face and Prudence met me for the first time in the bedroom. . . .
> I began to see that Prudence was going to be a bridge between my isolation from my surroundings because of my blindness, and from the general public. I realised that she was going to provide a talking point for people who wanted to help cheer me on my way but who, without the interest in a dog, would have been too shy to speak. . . . All these little episodes I found delightful and without realizing it I was altering and becoming a happy and relaxed person again. (Hickford, 1973, pp. 52, 68, 80)

One of the common misconceptions is that the dog is in control and the blind person's only responsibility is that of hanging on to the harness until the destination is reached. On the contrary, the blind person must be in control, knowledgeable of the route to the destination, and aware at all times of the immediate environment. Interaction with objects or landmarks in the environment may be more limited than with the use of a cane as the dog will, without the master's knowledge, frequently circumvent an obstacle.

On occasion the dog may be temporarily or permanently incapacitated. If the dog is ill, for example, the blind person must temporarily use another mode of travel. The working life of a dog is estimated to be from eight to twelve years, after which the owner must train with a new dog. The necessity of giving up a familiar and dependable working companion can be traumatic.

> Then it emerged that Paddy, her old dog, had had to be retired early because of illness, and had gone to friends near Dotty's home. "It's so *awful*," she went on, "to have left Paddy behind and to come for another dog. I feel I've betrayed her." (Hocken, 1977, p. 37)

Electronic Travel Aids

Electronic travel aids are not presently widely utilized as a mode of mobility for the visually impaired; however, as technological advances in our society become more commonplace, their potential will be more fully realized. Historically, some of the first devices came into being as adaptations of sensory instruments developed for use in the armed forces during World War II. Although several military obstacle detectors appeared to have possible implications for use by blind individuals, the first major apparatus manufactured exclusively for the visually impaired traveler was the Ultrasonic Aid or "Torch" developed in New Zealand.

Presently, training programs conducted by orientation and mobility specialists are limited to instruction in the utilization of four devices: the Russell Pathsounder, the Mowat Sensor, the Sonicguide, and the Laser Cane. The first three are normally used as supplements to the cane and operate by converting ultrasonic energy to feedback in the form of auditory information (Sonicguide), tactile or vibratory information (Mowat Sensor), or both (Pathsounder). The Sonicguide is the more complex mechanism and can determine range, laterality, and characteristics of objects encountered. The Laser Cane, in contrast, has its mechanics built into the cane itself and projects its feedback by converting energy from a light source (laser beams) into simple auditory and tactile information. These devices provide additional information that can be incorporated into the user's mental map of the environment. Unfortunately, most of the electronic travel aids are too expensive for widespread use.

Some visually impaired persons choose to travel without the use of any of the travel modes described above. This is understandable when they have sufficient residual vision to make this possible or when they are in familiar settings of home, classroom, or office where other safety techniques can be employed. Many low vision people have learned to travel by using visual clues from their environment, as distorted or limited as these are. Some of these clues may include color, contrast, direction of light source, or visual landmarks. Some low vision persons have learned adaptive behaviors such as the use of sunglasses for light sensitive individuals or the development of a constant scanning of the environment for the person with tunnel vision.

However, low vision individuals whose ability to function visually varies from one setting to the next may find travel difficulties fluctuating from easy to impossible. People with night blindness may function fairly well with adequate lighting but find travel extremely difficult at night or in dimly lit rooms unless they employ one of the travel techniques described above. The unpredictable nature of low vision is a source of inner conflict and turmoil (see Chapter 9).

There are some visually impaired persons who refuse to use a travel aid because they reject the symbolism of blindness that the aid represents. Refusal to utilize a travel aid reveals their feelings about themselves and may result in a risk to their personal safety. For example, a low vision person may choose to follow another pedestrian because he is able to track brightly colored clothing, but the pedestrian, never realizing that he is serving as a guide, may weave through congestion and leave the visually impaired person stranded. The rejection of the cane and its consequences are described by Mehta.

> I stood there, running my hand up and down my new long, thin cane, with a fancy strap instead of a handle at the top. I took the two

ends of the cane in my hands, and putting my foot at the center, pulled hard and broke it in two. And flinging it back into the gutter, I walked rapidly toward the school building. . . .

Once—I believe it was the first week of my work—I had just got off the bus and, taking the back way, was walking rapidly toward the ice-cream plant. All of a sudden I felt the firm ground under my feet give. I was falling in empty space. . . . The time between walking off the edge and landing in the slushy manhole all doubled up did seem to be endless. It was not the numbing pain or the shock that I minded so much, but the screaming and fainting of an old woman, and crowd of people who gathered immediately, clicking their tongues, some remarking that blind people should never be allowed out on the streets alone, others admonishing me for not carrying a cane, and I all the time suffused with shame—shame about what people thought. (Mehta, 1957, pp. 260, 263)

With respect to nonpedestrian travel, most sighted individuals enjoy, value, and even take for granted the mechanized mobility of society as evidenced by cars, recreation vehicles, motorcycles, private planes, etc. Neither the dog nor the cane, as good as they are, provide the freedom of mobility to which society has become accustomed.

The necessity to preplan and arrange for motorized travel, especially when public transportation is not available, has its effect on limiting the quality of a wide range of experiences and on a person's feelings of dependence. Furthermore, in a society where driving has become a significant milestone for the maturing adolescent, especially for boys, the inability to drive may raise questions about one's sex role identity. David, in the following excerpt, began to work through some of these feelings at the early age of seven.

We were driving along a narrow country lane when he began, "Will I be able to do this myself? Drive, I mean?"

There must be truth in answers to serious questions, so I answered, "No, David." . . .

"Then what am I going to do?"

I explained as nonchalantly as I could manage that it would in any case be a very long time before he was old enough to drive. This was not enough. He questioned, he queried. At last he sat, and I suggested that he would then have lots of friends who would drive for him. . . .

"All right," he said, "that'll do." He thumped his hand on the seat. "But it'll be my car." (Lunt, 1965, pp. 58-59).

The adult who prior to blindness had been driving frequently expresses the sentiment that giving up driving is one of the more painful deprivations resulting from loss of sight. Many adults, whether adventitiously or congenitally blind, express a frustration regarding the necessity of relying on others for transportation.

> Probably more important than earning one's own living is having the ability to move about at will. . . . To have to ask a friend or a busy member of the family to go along on the simplest of errands is more humiliating than most seeing people realize and humiliation brings with it a deep resentment at one's lot. (Irwin, 1955, p. 169)

A strong relationship exists between a blind person's ability to travel independently and his self-esteem, as is illustrated throughout the biographical sketches used in this section. Welsh (1980), an experienced Orientation and Mobility specialist, observed that "the lack of independent travel may lead to increased dependency, isolation, hopelessness, and a poor self-concept. . . . On the other hand, success in independent travel tasks, even at the beginning levels, can bring about an improved self-concept, a greater sense of independence, and improved motivation for other tasks" (p. 469).

IMPLICATIONS FOR READING AND WRITING

Most people in today's society are bombarded by the written word on every side: from private letters to street signs, from paperbacks to cereal boxes, from billboards to comic books, from store posters to classroom chalkboards, from assembly instructions to newspapers. The visually impaired population has potential access to some of the tremendous array of written word through one or more of a variety of modalities. Although braille is bulky, awkward, and slow (100 wpm), it is the best system for reading and writing for the blind thus far devised (Tuttle, 1972).

> Those of us who learn braille in middle life will always find it a slow and irritating substitute for visual reading. But every infuriating dot of it is worth a fortune! (Blackhall, 1962, p. 102)

Unfortunately, braille requires an intermediary (another

person between the printed word and the blind person) with knowledge of the braille code and specialized equipment to transcribe the printed page into braille.

Still more print is made available to the visually impaired by means of recordings. Like braille, access to print through recordings requires an intermediary with knowledge of format and recording equipment to read the material aloud. While audio reading is faster than braille (175-300 wpm), the processes of studying technical material—referencing, skimming, and scanning—are less efficient (Tuttle, 1981b). Lightweight and portable recording devices permit "writing" or taking notes, although indexing, storing, and retrieving these notes is awkward.

Although many low vision persons can use regular print and standard writing tools without modification or simply by holding the material closer, some require large print, large type, or optical magnifiers. Even greater magnification can be achieved through the use of closed circuit televison readers or other electronic visual aids. With the exception of large type, which requires a typist, these reading methods provide the visually impaired person with direct access to print (without an intermediary).

More recently, some highly sophisticated yet expensive electronic devices have shown promise. The optacon ($4,000-$5,000) converts the shape of the print letter into a vibrating image felt under the index finger. It provides direct access to print (not script) with moderate to slow reading rate. The Kurzweil Reader (in excess of $20,000) uses computer technology and synthetic speech to electronically "read aloud" any printed material placed face down on its reading platform. Paperless braille word processers ($5,000-$10,000) use electronic impulses to code and store braille on standard audio cassettes that can subsequently be retrieved and displayed on a single line of electronically activated metal pins forming the braille. It becomes a braille terminal when interfaced with other electronic equipment having print displays.

When an intermediary person is required to make reading

material available to the blind person as in braille or talking books, the range of choice is much more limited because of the mandatory selectivity process and, on occasion, censorship.

Apart from these occasional personal prejudices on the part of the transcriber, one does still sometimes come across other instances of unwillingness to allow the blind reader the same freedom of choice as is enjoyed by the sighted one, though this is not nearly so marked as was once the case. With the dwindling of the century-old conviction that an affliction as terrible as blindness must be regarded as just punishment for sin, the tendency to limit the reading of the blind to improving books has almost died out — at least I hope it has, though I can't help remembering that when I first went to the Braille Library in Melbourne to arrange about having lessons, I was told that my own most successful novel, *A Warning to Wantons* had not been considered "nice" enough to be fit for circulation among the blind. What most annoyed me about this episode was the impossibility of protest, for I was convinced that would be ascribed to the hurt vanity of the author and not to the outraged indignation of the reader furious at the idea that any more censorship should be applied to the reading of the blind than was applied to the reading of the sighted. (Mitchell, 1964, p. 65)

The selection process and the time lag involved in making the reading materials available to the visually impaired pose a problem for one desiring to remain current in a specific or specialized field. Although some general periodicals are available, many specialized periodicals and local newspapers are not. Some communities have established radio reading services to help meet this need. In a community where a radio reading service was not available, Graeme Edwards dealt with the problem in his own way.

The broadcasts made life busier for me and were certainly the most interesting part of my week's work. They brought new problems. From now on I had to keep up not only with the news, but with as much comment as I could find.... I realized I would have to hire readers two or three times a week and that journalists would be the most valuable for what I wanted. (Edwards, 1962, p. 77)

When all else fails, many blind persons secure the services of a person either paid or volunteer to read the desired print material. However, one sacrifices a certain amount of intimacy or privacy when sharing one's private mail with a reader.

> I regard the need of having to deal with so much of my correspondence through a third person as one of the most crushing blows to my privacy, directly attributable to blindness. The normal excitement of opening a letter from a long distance, except from a blind friend, switches to frustration, and sometimes agitation. I have to find somebody to do me the favour of reading it aloud, and if I think it will be a really personal letter I may have to wait some time before I find the person with whom I want to share it. . . . I have not worked out how to handle the situation when someone with me offers to read a letter from a mutual friend, if I think there might be some confidential passage in it. At least I would like to know what my friend has said before I pass it around. (Edwards, 1962, pp. 89-90)

Of course, privacy in reading one's personal mail is retained when family members and friends take the time to learn braille and use it in their notes and correspondence. When this happens, the self-esteem of the blind person is enhanced because it represents a respect for his dignity and worth as an individual.

> So much of my privacy has gone that there is a heightened joy in having something of my very own. One of my sisters lives in Devon and I remember, with pleasure and humility, that it was from her I received my first letter in braille. She had taken the trouble to learn the system and had bought a braille writing frame in order that she could write to me in my own language. This was better than all the rivers of grief, better than condolences, better than occupational therapy. This was that kind of sympathy for which no words will ever be found, that kind of understanding which enables people to touch hands, though they are a thousand miles apart. (Blackhall, 1962, p. 166)

Although the use of braille, large print, or magnifiers may enhance reading and writing abilities, some visually impaired people reject them because their use makes them feel self-conscious and different. The rejection of coping techniques and adaptive behaviors reveals much regarding the person's feelings about himself, his blindness, and his self-esteem.

Vocational Implications

Even with all the recent social and legislative focus on

civil rights for the handicapped, most blind adults have not experienced full and equal assimilation into the work force. In the first place they experience high unemployment (Kirchner and Peterson, 1980; Lowenfeld, 1975). Second, those who enter the job market are frequently underemployed, employed in positions utilizing less than optimum qualifications and abilities, and frequently underpaid (Scholl et al., 1969). In the third place, once a blind person is employed, he experiences discriminatory practices that inhibit normal advancement. After receiving his degrees from Oxford and Yale, unable to find a college teaching position, and being refused factory jobs, Russell illustrates the devastating effects of extreme underemployment when he was left with no alternatives but to accept employment in a sheltered workshop.

> After all these years . . . to have to go back into a shelter! Since I had left the Institute I had been in open competition with sighted people, and now, when it really mattered, when I had a wife to look after and a whole new life to build, I was being forced back inch by inch, day by day, into the world from which I thought I had broken free.
> Worst of all was being reminded of the shame—not the shame of defeat, but the deep and insidious shame of blindness. Being forced back into the workshop was to be reminded all over again of my inadequacy, all over again to clench my fists in impotent rage, to feel all over again the hot tears scald my cheeks. (Russell, 1962, pp. 286-287)

There are many reasons for this unfortunate state of affairs. Rusalem (1972) listed three common barriers to employment:

> the lack of general readiness on the part of the blind person to use the tools and techniques that have been devised to overcome some of the effects of blindness, the lack of creativity and imagination on the part of some rehabilitation workers who tend to cast blind workers into stereotyped vocational roles, and the lack of sufficient systematic occupational research to devise improved means of performing more jobs without sight (p. 22).

A fourth barrier is to be found in the prejudices or misinformation held by employers, resulting in a reluctance to hire a blind person (Lowenfeld, 1975).

> But when Bob tells the business man that he doesn't want money—

he wants a chance for a blind person to earn it—that's another matter. Even though the employer has read stories in the newspapers about blind persons working in factories, his hair stands on end when he thinks of a blind person in *his* factory. In his mind's eye he sees a blind man getting caught in the machinery, running into things on the way to the rest room, and throwing his entire factory into panic and confusion. (Moore, 1960, p. 149)

Another contributing factor according to Rusalem (1972) is that some blind persons are poorly prepared to enter the job market. "Theoretically graduates of schools and classes for the blind should be ready for vocational training or placement without delay. Not infrequently, however, despite secondary school prevocational experiences, such students emerge with their academic abilities clearly defined, but with many questions about their vocational interests and capacities" (p. 151). He felt that because many schools fail to assess visually impaired student's interests, aptitudes, and potentialities comprehensively, they leave school lacking clearly defined vocational plans for the future.

Career education for the visually impaired begins in early primary grades and continues throughout school. Elements of this program include role playing, job behaviors, job information, job exploration, part-time jobs, job seeking skills, job training, job tryouts, and vocational evaluation. The process is not much different from that for the sighted; however, it requires more careful and systematic planning and sequencing of activities provided jointly by the special education teacher, the school counselor, and the vocational rehabilitation counselor. With adequate educational opportunities and a wide range of experiences, a blind teen-ager can mature vocationally without any more guidance than his sighted peers receive (VanderKolk, 1981).

For the individual blinded between the ages of 20 and 60, there is usually a disruption in employment. His initial preoccupation is with the development of some personal adjustment skills in travel, communication, and techniques of daily living, after which employment needs once again become salient.

Historically, blind people were counseled into a narrow

range of specific jobs such as broom-making, chair-caning, piano-tuning, etc., with many becoming stereotypically associated with blind people. In time, more and more blind people demonstrated competence and abilities in a greater and greater variety of jobs.

> There was a time when agencies and individuals attempted to compile lists of pursuits in which blind people are active. With the advent of organized rehabilitation this practice was abandoned because those concerned with placement discovered practically from day-to-day new possibilities of employment which suited an individual client and were not included in any of the compiled job lists. (Lowenfeld, 1975, p. 161)

> First I had to find out what I could do, then convince people who were not used to blindness that the difficulties were not insurmountable, and finally, having once got the chance, to carry out what I had claimed I could manage. (Edwards, 1962, p. 173)

Fortunately, the current trend is more toward tailoring the job to the blind person, his interests, and abilities rather than tailoring the blind person to the available jobs. The more that a person's interests and abilities are matched to the demands of his employment, the greater is the likelihood for job satisfaction since job satisfaction, one's employment, and one's self-esteem are inextricably intertwined.

> That night I went home happier than ever. I had made good on my first job.... This was a tremendous victory because it showed I was good for something after all, not just a sightless liability. (Sheppard, 1956, p. 47)

IMPLICATIONS FOR RECREATION

For many visually impaired, leisure-time activities take on special significance. With adequate training and opportunities, they provide many hours of personal satisfaction, creative productivity, and social companionship. Recreational activities cover a broad spectrum of hobbies, collections, arts and crafts, games, sports, and other outdoor activities such as mountain climbing.

> I do not climb mountains in order to break records of height or altitude. Those things do not interest me. I do it because I love the

beauty and simplicity of a way of living which brings confidence,
which confirms resolution and calls for courage. (Richard, 1966, p. 17)

Lacking the opportunity for visual observation and imitation, many visually impaired individuals are not sufficiently familiar with some of these activities to know their potential for personal enjoyment. With sufficient training to assure full appreciation of each activity, blind children and adults are enabled later to make intelligent decisions about whether to engage in these activities. With the exception of some team sports, most of these activities require little or no modification for the visually impaired. As a result, blind persons are able to participate along with sighted individuals. For some sports that are specially adapted (such as golf or bowling), local, state, and national events are available for those who want to compete with other blind individuals.

A common observation, especially among the adventitiously blind, is that of having too much time, of being bored, of having nothing to do.

There was, however, much enforced idleness throughout the day—
a new and discomfiting experience for one who had heretofore been
so active. (McCoy, 1963, p. 42)

Recently blinded adults seem surprised sometimes to discover they can still enjoy previous forms of entertainment such as dancing, concerts, and movies. Some parents, spouses, and friends unwittingly fall into the trap of permitting the blind person to retreat into a world of radio, television, and recordings. In moderation, these can be excellent forms of entertainment, but they should never become the sole source lest the blind person withdraw into his own fantasy world.

Through radio I became a mad fan of international cricket and big
football series.... Like blindness itself, broadcasting tended to have
the effect of driving me into my own company perhaps too much and
separating me from the lives of the rest of the household. This reached
an extreme during one short phase, which fortunately my parents
discouraged. (Edwards, 1962, pp. 13-14)

Finally, one of the greatest values of recreational activities is the opportunity they provide a blind person to interact socially with sighted individuals as together they engage in a common activity. (Kelley [1981] provides guidelines for integrated recreational activities.) Unfortunately, too many agencies for the blind foster and encourage segregated recreational programs far beyond the time required for rehabilitative training in recreation (Lowenfeld, 1975).

> Successful recreation, then, is more than the selection and adaptation of leisure time activities. It is part of the total social adjustment of the individual. . . . One may be enticed into partici- pating in many activities and still remain unhappy and poorly adjusted. It is not that we need more recreational activities, but that we need the right kind conducted under conditions that lead to growth in social adjustment for the visually handicapped individual. (Buell, 1951, p. 12)

The values, goals, and benefits of recreation are the same whether the person is blind or sighted. "The primary purpose of recreation is to provide programs and services that make possible individualized recreative experiences— experiences characterized by feelings of mastery, achieve- ment, exhilaration, acceptance, success, personal worth, and pleasure" (Carter and Kelley, 1981, p. 65).

SUMMARY

The direct effects of a visual loss have been discussed with respect to the practical impact on day-to-day operations in the areas of personal and home management, travel, read- ing and writing, vocation, and recreation. For either con- genitally blind or adventitiously blind persons, their level of self-esteem is affected by the extent to which there is a lack or loss of independence in any of these areas. Rather than being permanent, most of the negative consequences are temporary until remediated by training in the use of adaptive aids, devices, and techniques. It follows, therefore, that the impact of blindness on self-esteem should be of a temporary nature, although nonetheless devastating. The next chapter will deal with the psychosocial implications of blindness.

Chapter 3

PSYCHOSOCIAL IMPLICATIONS
OF BLINDNESS

T here is no special psychology of blindness, no personality unique to blind persons (Foulke, 1972; Kirtley,
1975; Lowenfeld, 1981; Schulz, 1980; Sommers, 1944). Personality traits and life adjustment patterns are as varied
among the visually impaired as among the seeing.

> No new or special psychological principles are required to explain
> the behavior of the blind or attitudes toward blindness: certain
> established principles of general psychology are fully adequate to
> this task.... The difference of the blind lies solely in their
> experience of visual deficit and certain behavioral limitations
> inherent in that deficit. (Kirtley, 1975, pp. ix-x)

The psychological impact of low vision and blindness can
best be understood within the sociological framework. Low
vision persons tend to have more difficulty establishing
their personal identity because of their ambiguous, poorly
defined role within a sighted world. The first part of this
chapter will deal with some sociological dynamics of vision
loss including attitudes toward blindness. Then some concerns within the psychological domain will be discussed
with a brief introduction to an adjustment model. Finally,
some of the literature regarding the self-concept of the
visually impaired will be reviewed.

SOCIOLOGICAL IMPLICATIONS

The quality and characteristics of the social interaction

between a blind and a sighted person are determined by the capacities and attitudes of each. First to be considered are some of the direct social consequences of the condition of blindness. As is so often true, broad generalizations always have their exceptions. Thus, the application of the following tendencies to any specific person must be guarded. Furthermore, many of the sociological consequences are temporary until techniques are learned that remediate or circumvent the difficulty.

Immature and Egocentric Behavior

Visually impaired children and young adults tend to be more socially immature and remain more egocentric longer than their sighted peers. Unless countermanded, the restriction to nonvisual stimuli inhibits the development of the ability to view the world from another's perspective. Recently blinded adults as well tend to regress into more egocentric attitudes and behaviors. Preoccupation with the many new adjustment and coping problems precipitated by blindness prevents one from reaching out to others.

> I wanted to be taken care of, read to, provided for. I wanted her to arrange for new lighting, to discuss my thesis with me, to give me advice on my counseling efforts. My blindness blinded me to Charlotte's needs: *she* wanted to be cared for, even by the likes of me. (Potok, 1980, p. 86)

A person who is visually impaired is sometimes self-conscious. Congenitally blind children, not understanding vision and unable to predict when they can or cannot be seen, are uncertain about when they are being observed. Newly blind youth and adults often express the feeling they are constantly being watched. In either case, the self-conscious feelings may result from the realization that, as blind persons using specialized coping skills and aids, they are seldom able to blend into the crowd, to remain anonymous.

> About me I heard the scratch of pens on paper as students took notes on the professor's lecture. I was too self-conscious to put my Braille slate on the table before me and start punching. It would attract

everybody's attention. I dreaded being looked upon as different. With a supreme effort, I forced my pride to bend. I put a sheet of heavy Braille paper in my slate and began rattling away with my stylus. The tick, tick, tick, as the point pierced the paper, resounded throughout the room. My ears grew hot. I felt as conspicuous as a snore in church. It was hard work punching through the heavy paper. My arm tired. I lost the continuity of the professor's thought—at least I thought I did. I discovered later that he didn't have any continuity. (Ohnstad, 1942, p. 185)

Isolation and Withdrawal

Someone who is visually impaired has a tendency to be more frequently socially isolated or to have feelings of isolation and detachment. He is not always able to choose his companion for conversation, often needing to wait to be spoken to first. In a group, he frequently finds it difficult to know when comments are directed to him. He is less able to observe the nonverbal undertones of social interaction. Many times the isolation results from the sighted person's uncertainty about approaching a blind person.

> It is not easy for a seeing person to realize how difficult it is for a blind person to strike the correct balance in a room full of people. If I talk too much, I will certainly make myself conspicuous. On the other hand, if I sit like a bump on a log, I can expect to be ignored. But I cannot make advances to people unless they first come and speak to me, and thoughtful people realize that this is so. Yet anyone unaccustomed to being with the blind may not realize how powerless I am under the circumstances. (Dahl, 1962, p. 139)

As with so many of the sociological problems mentioned in this section, it requires ingenuity and advanced planning to circumvent the problem, in this case the isolating factor of blindness.

> Dating was hard work, requiring planning, attention to detail, persistence, and patience. If I met someone I thought might be interesting and if I learned, say, that we were going to have a class together the following semester, I'd start plotting how to arrange for our seats accidentally to be in proximity. I had to develop nonchalant ways of finding out what interesting girls were sitting around me, then figure out how to strike up conversations, each of which might take a day or two of planning. Before going too far, I'd always check with some guy I trusted: "Is she good looking?" They'd usually give me

straight answers. . . .

In short, dating was never a relaxed, enjoyable business, but a great labor to be worked at. Still, I was determined to succeed. I was always worried about the last date, planning ways to refine this or that on the next one. I've often said to Cheri that until we were married I never appreciated girls. All of a sudden I was free at last to relax and just make friends. (Hartman and Asbell, 1978, pp. 77-78)

The difficulties involved in overcoming social isolation may be so overwhelming that the blind person simply gives up and physically withdraws.

I was never deliberately ostracized by the students. It was just that with a handful of exceptions, they made no attempt to draw me into their circles. Because I found no real friends in the Lowell House dining room, I very rarely went there. I would buy one meal a day, usually at Elsie's Cafe, and take it to my room, there to eat alone. I have never felt before or since the stark, continuous loneliness I experienced in that room. (Sullivan and Gill, 1975, p. 110)

The temptation to withdraw physically, socially, and emotionally contributes to a potentially active phantasy life, which is detached from the real world (Cutsforth, 1951; Schulz, 1980).

Like many shy, imaginative children, he had built his own little world, and he could enter it at will and leave everything else outside. This withdrawing into himself was heightened by his blindness and became one of the most serious obstacles to overcome. (Henderson, 1954, p. 73)

Passivity and Dependency

A person who is visually impaired tends to be more passive, less assertive. Unable to immediately perceive alternative courses of action, such as which door to enter an unfamiliar building, he is more frequently limited to the one first discovered. Frequently, decisions are made for him without consulting him, depriving him of the opportunity to develop and practice his ability to make choices. He is frequently less able to observe or anticipate situations that permit him to initiate or exercise social courtesies on his own such as picking up a dropped object for someone. Although most attempts to be more assertive can be successful given proper information, there are times when these attempts backfire.

> "Hey, Hal, you're never going to pick up a girl just standing there," shouted Ben as he danced by me. "Assert yourself, dammit; just wade into this mob and ask someone to dance." . . .
>
> "Pardon me, I wonder if you'd care to dance," I shouted to the individual standing next to me.
>
> "No thanks, I'm heterosexual at the moment. But listen, if I should ever decide to swing the other way, I'll be sure to look you up," boomed a deep male voice.
>
> I stood there, wishing that the floor would open and swallow me. (Krents, 1972, p. 197)

Hartman, while studying to be a medical doctor, was able to make his own decisions after soliciting the information required.

> Wayne would often serve as a pair of eyes. He was good at it. Learning to depend on him for certain observations while reserving independence in decision making was valuable training for me. In medicine, doctors depend constantly on other people's observations—X rays, electrocardiograms, lab tests, all sorts of nurses' reports—and I have to rely on the reports of others a little more than most, yet make my own decisions. (Hartman and Asbell, 1978, p. 91)

Finally, less able to perceive the conditions for correct or appropriate behavior and unwilling to actually do something wrong, the visually impaired individual may unconsciously accept the motto that to do nothing is better than to do something wrong, to withdraw is better than to make a fool of oneself.

> At dances I'd sit absolutely petrified in case a boy asked me to be his partner. I was so scared I would make mistakes or not be able to follow what he was doing. . . .
>
> I remember one particularly terrible occasion when a boy left me standing in the middle of the dance floor after the music stopped, and I could hear everyone else moving away. I felt a sense of space opening up around me as the noise of the dancers receded to the edges of the hall. I pretended to tidy my hair but inside I was panicking until I heard someone approach. Angela had come to rescue me.
>
> After that I gave up going to dances because it was such a trial. (Hocken, 1977, pp. 17-18)

A person who is visually handicapped is more frequently

placed in a position of dependency on others. This severely interferes with the natural drive toward self-sufficiency and autonomy, the drive to be found on equal footing with others.

> Apart from all these considerations there was a deeper reason why I did not want to employ a secretary. I have spoken already of my belief that parasitism is a terrible and destructive force, and after my sight began to fail it did not take me long to learn that there is among the sighted a strongly held belief that loss of sight must inevitably involve loss of all independence, that only with the help of the sighted can a blind person live and work. This belief is the harder to combat because it is partly true. Some loss of independence there must be with the loss of sight. (Mitchell, 1964, p. 22)

Some blind children and young adults who have developed a pattern of accepting help begin to confuse "those who help" with "friends." Their friends, they reason, should help, and those who help are their friends. This dependent relationship on "friends" tends to deteriorate with time. This will be discussed further in Chapters 4 and 9. By anticipating the problem, Krents was able to avoid the confusion between helper and friend.

> My only contact with females was the twenty hours a week that I spent with my staff of readers. As far as I was concerned, there were not two but three sexes—males, females, and readers. I took a practical stand when it came to my relationships with the girls who read my textbooks to me. For one thing, you don't tend to get much work done if you're dating the girl who's reading to you. And for another, if you break up with your reader or if she breaks up with you, kablam! not only have you lost a reader, but much more importantly you've lost two hours a week of study. (Krents, 1972, p. 124)

Inadequate Social Role Models

Because social behaviors and attitudes are learned by observation and imitation, a person who is visually impaired finds it difficult to emulate the available role models. The number, range, and variety of observations are more limited, and the opportunities for participating in social situations more restricted (Scott, 1969b). Blind persons, especially children, have little basis for comparison and so do not

realize that some of their behaviors are socially unacceptable. Some of these are self-stimulating mannerisms commonly known as "blindisms," which when extinguished
must be replaced with more socially accepted behaviors.

In addition to the restricted opportunities to model social
behavior, the low incidence of blindness limits the number
of blind persons available to model adaptive or coping
behaviors. However, not all blind persons exhibit behaviors
and attitudes that should be modeled.

> Although my mother was concerned about my cruel treatment of
> him [his blind tutor], she was even more concerned about the effect
> that his own attitude about his blindness was having upon me. My
> parents had always taught me to believe that I was a normal, well-
> adjusted child who just happened not to see. Mr. J., who had been
> educated in blind schools before going to college, believed that an
> acceptance of the tremendous limitations that blindness imposed
> could not be acknowledged too early in life. (Krents, 1972, p. 111)

Fox, on the other hand, received strength and inspiration
from blind friends he had met at the rehabilitation center.

> The second big step in the building up of my morale was meeting
> the other blind students.... Their attitude toward life and the ease
> with which they carried on the business of living, helped me a lot....
> Here was living proof that blindness was not an unconquerable
> handicap. They made blindness seem a natural thing.... I still have
> moments of depression, but when I do, I can always snap out of it by
> remembering those blind men and women and the things they are
> doing. Surely if they can find happiness and success, I can do the same
> thing. (Fox, 1946, pp. 185, 188)

In spite of knowing socially appropriate behavior, sometimes blind persons find themselves in awkward or embarrassing predicaments. Some can be anticipated and thus
avoided; yet not all potentially embarrassing situations can
or should be avoided. To do so would foster further isolation
and detachment. It is far better to learn to laugh at
embarrassing situations that are beyond one's control.

> My worst embarrassment happened during an excited babble of
> voices when I afforded a convention its greatest laugh by kissing the
> wrong woman. What amused my friends the most was the fact that
> instead of kissing my sister-in-law, I had smacked the one who had
> said many unkind things about me and my work. (Fries, 1980, p. 372)

Stereotypic Attitudes

Persons who are visually impaired encounter a wide divergence of predominantly negative attitudes toward blindness (Lukoff et al., 1972). Many of the stereotypic misconceptions have a depressing effect on the self-esteem of blind persons especially when these attitudes are held by parents, teachers, rehabilitation workers, and even the blind person himself. People become the role they are expected to play (Gergan, 1971). Congenitally blind children come to accept these negative attitudes without question. Adventitiously blind persons carry with them into blindness many of these attitudes previously acquired.

> The world's notions about the blind are fixed and capable of appraisal, and off hand I can think of no people who are more unremittingly subjected to a body of notions about them than the blind. . . . And upon examination, we find that all of the reactions in an individual which we unthinkingly ascribe to the fact of blindness are caused instead by the world's attempt to impose its fixed notions on him. A man has these notions imposed on him, before he loses his sight as well as after. Such notions are not born in us but educated into us; they are picked up along with our deepest and most fundamental concepts of what makes happiness or unhappiness. After blindness has struck, although the individual may have discovered for himself the falsity of the concepts, society goes on imposing its notions sometimes to the point of defeating him. (Chevigny, 1946, p. 81)

Many have studied the sociological origins of common misconceptions and stereotypes that are held regarding the blind (Barker et al., 1953; Kirtley, 1975; Lowenfeld, 1975; Lukoff et al., 1972; Monbeck, 1973). These common attitudes are couched in several beliefs about blind persons:

1. inferior, subhuman, helpless, and useless

> There is amusement, too, when a new acquaintance on going to the china closet exclaims that the dishes are clean. Did she fancy that I ate off dirty plates and drank out of unwashed cups? Funny idea. (Bretz, 1940, p. 191)

2. pitiable, miserable, and wretched

> Some of them pitied us, and that's one thing none of us could stand. Some of them gave us the feeling that the only reason they had for spending their time and money on us was so they could brag to their

friends about how much they were doing for the poor, wounded servicemen. (Fox, 1946, pp. 138-139)

3. to be feared, avoided, and rejected especially in intimate relationships
4. emotionally and sexually maladjusted
5. associated with death
6. paying for previous sin, immoral, and evil
7. to be ridiculed for stupidity, impaired understanding, and other generalized incapacities

> Since blind people find it very difficult to keep track of what is happening around them, some of their friends suspect that something more than our eyesight has failed us. They think that in some way we have become mentally affected, and they treat us as if we were childish or worse.
>
> I have frequently been present when people who mean no harm whatever have made it clear that they feel I have no capacity to take part in a conversation. They ignore me entirely. (Dahl, 1962, p. 140)

8. unemployable

> [Hiram's father shared his concerns with Fries:]
> "Hiram had just lost his sight, and it was beyond my comprehension to know how he could ever be happy and successful at anything without being able to see." (Fries, 1980, p. 149)

9. unapproachable with comfort or ease
10. living in constant darkness or blackness

> Slogans such as one popular in Australia, "seventy years in darkness" have all helped to build up a pathetic public picture of the blind. (Edwards, 1962, p. 83)

11. to be tolerated, indulged, or excused
12. superhuman, or supernaturally endowed or compensated

> "I remember one time when Mable was proof-reading for the Commission, a man who worked upstairs stopped her in the hall one day and asked if blind people ever sin. Mable said of course they did, they were just like sighted people. And then later she found out he was losing his sight, and we thought he probably wanted to know if he was automatically going to become a saint when he could no longer see!" (Moore, 1960, p. 108)

13. reminders of everyone's vulnerability

14. deserving of sympathy, understanding, and respect
15. competent and capable.

These attitudes toward blind persons manifest themselves in and help to determine the behavior of an individual toward a person who is visually impaired. The behavior of others when interpreted and internalized by the blind person helps to mold and shape his self-concept. The behavior of the visually handicapped not only emerges from his self-concept but also influences the attitudes of those observing him. Baker (1973, p. 317) has illustrated the interrelationship between attitudes, behaviors, and self-concept as shown in Figure 3.

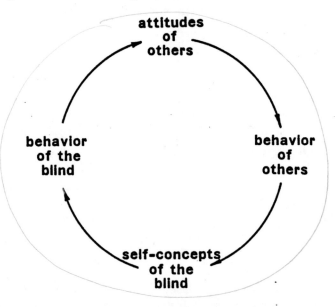

Figure 3. Interrelationship between Attitude, Behavior, and Self-concept. From Figure 1, "Socialization Process for the Blind" from "Blindness and Social Behavior: A Need for Research," by L.D. Baker in *New Outlook*, 1973, 67, 317. Reprinted with permission from the *New Outlook*, published by the American Foundation for the Blind.

The visually impaired person's behavior not only influences the attitudes of others toward himself but reflects directly back to his self-concept and self-esteem. How the blind person feels about himself, how he feels about blindness, and how he feels about the attitudes of others toward him are as important a determiner of his self-esteem as are the adaptive behaviors and coping skills he acquires.

The attitudes of others toward blindness and the self-regarding attitudes in one's self-concept can be changed, but not easily. Apparently knowledge alone, that is information about blindness by itself, is insufficient to stimulate significant attitude changes. (Bateman, 1962; Wyder, Wilson, and Frumkin, 1967). It also requires an experiential base, the opportunity to know and interact frequently over a period of time, for these attitudes to change.

Persons who are visually impaired often experience resistance to assimilation into society. Assimilation is more difficult when differences are perceived as significant (Wright, 1960). DeLevie (1966) found that persons who were disabled were perceived as profoundly different solely on the basis of the handicap. When individuals in society really come to know a blind person as more than just a casual acquaintance, blindness becomes insignificant and sometimes temporarily forgotten. The person is no longer *blind*, but a person who, among other things, happens to be blind.

> It is important for me to know that Oak Park has accepted me not as a blind person but as an individual who might have something to contribute to community life, and it is on this basis that I have been asked to participate in civic affairs. This acceptance has made it possible for me to keep looking forward and to progress, little by little. (Clifton, 1963, pp. 252-253)

Nonassimilation can also occur when the blind person himself perceives his differentness to be significant. Cholden, a psychiatrist, observed these feelings among the blind clients with whom he worked.

> While such feelings of uniqueness of emotions are not unusual in the sighted, I believe them to be much more common with the blind, because they are so limited in their ability to observe the emotional reactions of others. More than feeling that some fear or discomfort is specific for them, some of our clients feel that their emotions are mental abnormalities which serve to make them different from others. (Cholden, 1958, p. 37)

Some of the sociological difficulties just described are inherent in the condition of blindness; others are rooted in common attitudes found in society. The former can be remediated or circumvented by training in special techniques and by creative ingenuity. The latter cannot be resolved by legislation, as important as that is, or by demanding one's rights, as important as that may be, but rather by patient cultivation of personal relationships.

PSYCHOLOGICAL IMPLICATIONS

The psychological implications to be considered include the learning of concepts, abilities and school achievement, personality traits, and the process of adjusting with blindness. The cognitive and affective needs of persons who are visually impaired are the same as they are for all persons, and these needs are met in much the same way. A blind child is first of all a child, and his growth and development follow the same sequential pattern of development as that of a sighted child although in some areas his rate may be slower (Scholl, 1973). The slower rate of development is exemplified by the difficulties encountered in conceptualization.

Conceptualization

> She [the psychologist] gave Davey a tiny doll chair, and he did not know what it was. It was the first time he had held a chair in his hands, and we realized then that he had no real conception of the overall shape of a chair. He had sat on one, had touched the legs and the back, but he did not know how it all went together to make a chair. I was amazed at his agility with words and almost equally amazed at his ineptness with his hands. (Henderson, 1954, p. 111)

The properties and attributes of people, objects, and events are learned by interacting with one's physical and social environment. For most children, vision plays a dominant role in the conceptualization process. For the visually impaired child, the more severe the visual loss, the less he can depend on visual sensory data and the more he must rely on integrating information from the other senses, primarily tactile and auditory. While unimpaired vision enables a person to perceive the whole and then subsequently its parts and the relationship of the parts to each other and to the whole, the tactile-auditory process requires that a person, after examining the parts, integrate the parts into a mental whole. The latter conceptualization process is much less efficient and much more susceptible to deficient or incomplete concepts. "The misconceptions which can arise from fragmented and unrelated discoveries are nicely illustrated in the comment of a young blind child who on hearing a cow bellow asked his teacher, 'Which horn did she blow?'" (Chapman, 1978, pp. 20-21).

> One of the problems of a blind child is the fear of the unknown. Animals always gave me a sense of foreboding. Grandpa had four pigs and I kept asking to see them, but always when he was ready to put my hands on one of them, I drew back in fear. One day he laughed and told me he would let me "ride the pig to butcher". I stood and heard the pigs squealing as they caught them, and when Grandpa came to get me, I ran away. That night I felt the meat in the big stone jars. I was disappointed. I didn't think a pig looked like that. (Brown, 1958, p. 5)

Furthermore, conceptualization without vision has some inherent difficulties. Some objects and events are too large (Statue of Liberty), too tiny (amoeba), too far away (lunar eclipse), too dangerous (burning building), or too quick and unexpected (car accident) to permit careful nonvisual observations. The formulations and subsequent refinement of one's concepts require a variety of repeated experiences, whether first-hand or through pictures, television, movies, etc. Opportunities for a similiar range of reinforcing experiences are more limited for blind persons and require more careful planning. Napier (1973) recommended the use of actual objects, three-dimensional models, two-dimensional relief illustrations, each appropriately supplemented by verbal descriptions.

> One night we had a violent storm and a solitary pine tree keeled over and fell across the wild end of the garden, our wilderness.... The children were delighted. A tree they could get level with was something very special.... The interest was intense. "Does it go all the way to the sky? What does it hit on top? Who holds it up? Was it tired of

standing up and did it just let go?" These and many more questions
came and came again. We explored the root formation and stood in
the pit and I explained about the air and sky. (Lunt, 1965, p. 27)

Verbal descriptions by themselves provide an inadequate
base for concept formulation. Blind children who hear
words and then use them without the experiential base for
adequate understanding are engaging in "verbalism"
(Cutsforth, 1951). Most people engage in a certain amount of
verbalism: nuclear fission, moon walking, panning for gold,
etc. Unfortunately, blind children who have not been
encouraged to explore and interact with their environment
tend to exhibit more of this verbalizing behavior. A blind
child who has never been to the seashore may be able to talk
about "waves," "white caps," and "jelly fish" without an
adequate understanding of any of them.

The problem of verbalism is not unique to congenitally
blind children. The extent to which an adventitiously
blinded adult encounters new concepts but is content with
old experiences will determine how quickly he finds himself
living more and more in the past.

I know that the garden which I loved as a child and still remember
vividly is now an overgrown wilderness, but when I think of it I still see
it as it used to be. . . . Again, the faces of friends which I last saw clearly
about fifteen years ago have not changed for me though my reason
tells me that with the passing of time they must have changed. If
therefore the blind man in his efforts to keep in touch with the sighted
world leans too heavily on his recollections his efforts may create a
gulf rather than a bridge: he will be living in the past while they are
living in the present. (Mitchell, 1964, p. 148)

The potential for blind persons to gain an adequate understanding of people, objects, and events in their environment
including the self in relationship to that environment
remains intact. However, they frequently lack repeated,
first-hand, concrete experiences upon which to formulate
and validate clear hypotheses about the world around them.
"The effects of blindness modify some cognitive functions,
and this may have a retarding influence, more noticeable
during the preadolescent period. All this, however, does not
prevent normal achievement according to the individual's

capacity" (Lowenfeld, 1971b, p. 287).

Abilities and Achievements

It should be clear, then, that blindness in and of itself does not impair one's innate ability to process or manage sensory information intellectually. The limiting factor is the extent to which experiential interaction with the environment is improverished, thus inhibiting the blind person's ability to gather the greatest amount of alternative sensory information possible. "Vision is a medium or carrier of informational input, but not an indispensable medium" (Klein, 1962, p. 83).

There have been several approaches to the measurement of mental abilities in persons who are blind (VanderKolk, 1981). Some have focused on adapting tests standardized on the sighted while others have developed and normed tests specifically for the visually impaired population. When the verbal portions of standardized IQ tests for sighted were used, the measured intelligence of the visually impaired is distributed across the same normal range, some high, some low, but most clustering around the mean. There is no correlation between etiology of blindness and measured intelligence except in the cases of retinoblastoma and bilateral congenital anophthalmos (Lowenfeld, 1980). For some unknown reason, those with retinoblastoma tend to have higher measured IQ scores while those with anophthalmos tend to have lower scores.

With respect to academic achievement, there appears to be minimal age-grade retardation when achievement is measured with specially adapted tests for the visually impaired (Trismen, 1967). Although reading is slow, comprehension is maintained at grade level (Lowenfeld, Abel, and Hatlen, 1969). On the other hand, Stephens and Simpkins (1974) found as much as an eight-year lag in cognitive development among fourteen through eighteen year old congenitally blind children using a modified Piagetian assessment battery. With structured intervention, this lag is remediable (Stephens and Grube 1982). One would conclude that blind children have little difficulty with the rote learning involved in achievement measures, while the lag in abstract reasoning reflects restricted opportunities for environmental interaction, problem solving, and decision making. "The need for direct, concrete experience for blind children is of paramount importance. Direct physical experiences with the real object, total sensory and conceptual involvement with concrete objects, appropriate verbal interaction with other children and adults will help to give blind children a knowledge of the realities around them" (Swallow, 1976, p. 280).

Personality Traits

As previously discussed, there is no unique psychology of the blind, no unique set of psychological principles required to understand the behavior patterns of persons who happen to be blind. The essential "me" of the individual is the same before and after the trauma of blindness whether that trauma is the initial onset or subsequent confrontations with the social meaning of blindness.

> Of course no man is an island. No elephant is an island either. Just because I had suffered a transforming wound did not mean that I had at that instant also ceased the functions of life. This elephant's island was surrounded by others. I was still a husband, still a father, still a homeowner, still a workman, still a minister of Christ's church. All that I had been, I still was. (Kemper, 1977, pp. 68-69)

However, there are some personal, social, and emotional adjustment needs that are impacted by blindness. Blindness tends to aggravate or exacerbate latent or preexisting personality traits (Blank, 1957). The more dependent a person is, the more likely he will use blindness to rationalize even greater dependency. Someone who is by nature more independent may decide to either "do it himself" or do without and thus blame blindness for self-imposed restrictions. A nonconformist may use blindness as an excuse for eccentric behavior. A person employing self-protective defenses may use blindness as a convenient scapegoat for some personal inadequacies or failures unrelated to blindness (Wright, 1960). Unfortunately, the gullible, unenlightened "others" not only permit but encourage this form of rationalization.

The Adjusting Process

The process of adjusting to blindness and to the psychosocial impact of blindness follows the same pattern as adjusting to any severe trauma or significant change in one's life (Schulz, 1980). Although the process will be briefly introduced here, it will be described in greater detail in Section III. The stages or phases are sequential, not hierarchical, with a great deal of overlap between one phase and the next. Although the nature of the crisis for the congenitally blind may appear to be quite different from the trauma experienced by the adventitiously blind, the process of accommodating follows the same sequential pattern. Persons with any degree of restricted vision experience traumas directly attributable to their impaired vision and, after each trauma, to one degree or another proceed through the phases described as they search for self-acceptance and self-esteem.

TRAUMA, PHYSICAL OR SOCIAL. The physical or social trauma is the event or circumstance that precipitates the necessity for adjustment. For the congenitally blind, it may be the initial awareness that he is blind, that he is different. For the adventitiously blind, it may be the onset of blindness due to accident or disease. For both, it may be a recurring encounter with the social stigma of blindness.

SHOCK AND DENIAL. Feelings of unreality, detachment, and disbelief are common expressions during this phase. The shock is a form of psychic anesthesia enabling the self to incorporate subsequently the full significance of the tramatic impact bit by bit. Avoidance of the full significance of the trauma can also be accomplished by denying in one way or another that the source of the trauma exists.

MOURNING AND WITHDRAWAL. During this phase, the individual mourns or grieves for the generalized global loss of vision or the generalized global awareness of being "different." It is usually a time of self-pity when one withdraws from family and friends, a lonely time.

SUCCUMBING AND DEPRESSION. The individual begins to analyze, one by one, the perceived losses or inabilities regardless of whether they are realistic or not. This is the "I can't" phase. Although feelings of distress and doubt are common, in more extreme instances the emotional reactions of this phase may result in severe depression.

REASSESSMENT AND REAFFIRMATION. A reexamination of the meaning of life and purpose for living usually initiates a recovery. Sometimes reassessment precipitates a revision of one's values and goals, resulting in a reaffirmation of self and of life.

COPING AND MOBILIZATION. The reawakened desire to live life to the fullest and as independently as possible necessitates the development of techniques and strategies for coping with life's demands as a blind person. There is a willingness to identify oneself as blind and a desire to cope with the realities of blindness.

SELF-ACCEPTANCE AND SELF-ESTEEM. With the confidence that competence brings, the individual begins to develop or regain self-esteem as a person of dignity and worth. Rather than seeing himself as a blind person, he sees himself as a person with many characteristics and traits, only one of which is his blindness. He is comfortable with himself, he likes himself, he has acquired or regained self-acceptance and self-esteem.

A number of factors influence this adjustment process: age of onset, degree of vision, support of significant others, availability of professional services, etc. (see Chapter 9). Adjustment to blindness is not a static condition but rather a dynamic and fluid process, never ending.

Some perceive this adjustment process as arduous and difficult. "It is more difficult for a blind person than for a sighted to master his environment and thus feel adequate and competent to be an effective person" (Jervis, 1964, p. 52). The implication is that blind persons are more frequently frustrated than are the sighted, an assumption shared by Harley (1973) and Lowenfeld (1980).

However, Wright (1960) would disagree. "Though a disability may act as a barrier to the achievement of certain goals, the person in adjusting to this reality tends to alter his aspirations and way of life in such a way that oppressively frustrating situations are avoided" (p. 94). Thus, the blind person tends to reduce frustration by developing

adequate coping skills, by altering aspirations when necessary, and by occasionally altering his environment. However, this is not to imply that there are no frustrated blind
persons.

Adjustment to blindness, although perhaps difficult, is
nonetheless possible (Bauman, 1954a, 1969). Furthermore,
according to two studies there was no significant difference
in adjustment when comparing blind and sighted adolescents (Cowen et al., 1961; Sommers, 1944). Another significant finding of the latter two studies was the high correlation between understanding, accepting attitudes of significant others, particularly mothers, and positive adjustment
in visually imparied adolescents.

Self-concept and Self-esteem of Blind Persons

One of the key ingredients of good adjustment is a healthy
self-concept or positive self-esteem, the affective component
of self-concept. Fitts (1972) felt that self-concept was important to the rehabilitation or adjustment process in two
ways: "(1) the self-concept is a valid predictor of many
aspects of behavior; and (2) it is correlated with many other
variables (feelings, attitudes, interpersonal behavior, mental health) that may affect the rehabilitation performance"
(p. 9).

In several studies researchers have investigated the self-
concept of visually impaired children and youth but with
contradictory results. Early studies showed no essential
difference when comparing the self-concept of blind children and youth with that of comparable sighted people
(Jervis, 1959; Zunich and Ledwith, 1965). In both of these
studies, the visually impaired tended toward the extremes of
high and low self-ratings when compared with the sighted
children.

Meighan (1971) used the Tennessee Self-Concept Scale
with visually impaired secondary students in two residential
schools. He reported distinctly negative directions for all
measures of self-concept: identity, self-satisfaction, behavior,
physical self, moral-ethical self, personal self, family self,
and social self. More recently, Head (1979) using the same

instrument could not replicate the negative direction found in Meighan's study. In addition, Head found no significant difference when comparing the self-concept scores of visually impaired children across three educational settings: residential, resource, and itinerant. Coker (1979), using a different instrument with fourth through sixth-graders, concluded that "visually handicapped children in general were significantly happier and more satisfied than non-handicapped children as measured by Piers-Harris Children's Self-Concept Scale" (p. 73).

The contradictory findings may have resulted from the failure to recognize the dynamic, fluid nature of the adjusting process and its consequent interaction with the positive self-concept. Further research is needed to determine the effect on self-esteem of the constant demands for adjustment and readjustment occasioned by blindness and reactions to blindness. Blind persons who are struggling through the first four phases of the adjusting process (trauma, shock, mourning, and succumbing) experience a more negative overall self-esteem; those in the latter three phases (reassessment, coping, and self-acceptance) are in the process of rebuilding their self-esteem.

SUMMARY

This chapter has reviewed the sociological implications of blindness; the tendency toward immaturity, isolation, withdrawal, and passivity; as well as stereotypic attitudes held by both sighted and blind. It further reviewed the psychological implications of imparied vision, including concept development, abilities and achievements, personality traits, and the adjusting process. The sociological and psychological factors are all inherent in and intrinsic to but not necessarily requisites of blindness, and they may have a suppressing effect on one's sense of competence and self-esteem. When confronting physical or social traumas, an individual inevitably experiences some if not all of the adjusting phases enroute toward self-acceptance and self-esteem.

The development of healthy self-esteem enables a person

to respond and adapt to the demands of life in a confident manner. As a result, he earns the respect and admiration of others instead of pity and rejection. Section II will describe the internal and external factors that influence the development of one's self-esteem.

Section II
THE DEVELOPMENT OF
SELF-ESTEEM

Chapter 4

SOURCES OF SELF-ESTEEM, EXTERNALLY ORIENTED

T he social stigma of being disabled is learned (Goffman, 1963).

> The various attitudes and patterns of behavior that characterize people who are blind are not inherent in their condition but, rather, are acquired through ordinary processes of social learning. Thus, there is nothing inherent in the condition of blindness that requires a person to be docile, dependent, melancholy, or helpless; nor is there anything about it that should lead him to become independent or assertive. Blind men are made, and by the same processes of socialization that have made us all. (Scott, 1969a, p. 14)

The last chapter discussed that there is no unique psychology of blindness. The psychological principles involved in the dynamics of the development of one's self-concept or self-esteem among the sighted are equally applicable to persons who are blind. This unit will address the manner in which one's self-concept and self-esteem are acquired and explore the way blindness interacts with this process.

Because of the potentially negative direction of the interaction on self-esteem, both the external and internal sources of self-esteem need to be clearly understood. Delafield (1976) held the conviction that understanding the development of self-esteem is fundamental for the professional who works with blind persons.

> Most studies of the social adjustment process so far have been concerned with the role of significant others or with variables

unrelated to the individual. This has meant that the attitudes of
the blind person towards himself have been largely ignored....
Self-esteem is of central concern because of its dominant but
neglected influence on the adjustment process. (p. 67)

An individual's perception of his world and its demands,
coupled with his perceptions of his own abilities to cope with
those demands, are determinants of his behavior. In other
words, one's self-concept helps to determine how a person
adapts to his environment. "The way in which a man
conceives of himself will influence both what he chooses to
do and what he expects from life" (Gergan, 1971, p. 2).

SELF, SELF-CONCEPT, AND SELF-ESTEEM

Before discussing self-concept and self-esteem, it would be
helpful to understand what is meant by the word "self."
According to James (1890), the self is "the total sum of all
that he can call his" (p. 291). He further described the
constituents of the self as the "material self," bodily
appearance and appetites, love of home; the "social self,"
desire to please, to be noticed; and the "spiritual self," the
intellectual, moral, religious, and conscientious self. The
self encompasses both the "I" and the "me," both the
subject and the object of experience, both the knower and
the known.

The self, stable yet pliable, includes the "constant nature
of an individual plus all that is conditioned by time and
space and that is changeable. Self comes into being when ...
experiences are integrated into the uniqueness of the individual" (Wenkart, 1950, p. 91). The self evaluates life's
experiences and, as a general rule, assimilates and inte-
grates into itself that which is objective, positive, or reinforcing, while rejecting that which is harmful or inconsistent.

In the literature, the concept of self is closely aligned to
two other terms: personality and ego. The self has been
perceived as the nucleus of the personality. Personality "is
the dynamic organization within the individual of those
psycho-physical systems that determine his unique adjustments to his environment" (Allport, 1937, p. 48). Ego is "the

inferred self, that is, the personality structure that represents the core of decision-making, planning, and defensiveness" (Hamachek, 1971, p. 6). As can be seen, there is a great deal of overlap among these terms and, in common usage, they tend to be used interchangeably.

The perceptions and feelings an individual has about the self, whether realistic or not, cumulatively mold and shape the self-concept. According to Fitts (1967), "when we speak of the individual's self-concept we refer to the image, the picture, the set of perceptions and feelings which he has of himself" (p. 1). Thus both cognitive and affective dimensions are included in the self-concept.

Self-esteem is restricted more to the affective dimension of self-concept.

> By self-esteem we refer to the evaluation which the individual makes and customarily maintains with regard to himself: it expresses an attitude of approval or disapproval, and indicates the extent to which the individual believes himself to be capable, significant, successful, and worthy. In short, self-esteem is a *personal* judgment of worthiness that is expressed in the attitudes the individual holds toward himself. (Coopersmith, 1967, pp. 4-5)

Self-concept "may be either good or poor, may command esteem or be quite powerless to evoke it" (Stringer, 1971, p. 48). Self-esteem is part of, and emerges from, one's self-concept. The level of self-esteem is the evaluative component of the self-concept and presumes a fairly well-defined self-concept. Since a strong positive self-concept produces high self-esteem, in other words the one is a prerequisite for the other, when one speaks of good self-esteem, it presumes a healthy self-concept. Some synonyms for self-esteem include self-respect, self-worth, self-regard, self-acceptance, self-satisfaction, self-confidence, and self-love. Each of the notions represented by these terms can be perceived as ranging on a continuum from very high to very low.

The self, self-concept, and self-esteem are abstract, theoretical constructs that are not observable as physical entities but inferred from observing and interpreting verbal and nonverbal behaviors. Along with the inferred constructs are some assumptions about their properties and characteristics. The following principles have been synthesized from a review of the literature (Coopersmith, 1967; Fromm, 1947; Gergan, 1971; Hamachek, 1971; Horney, 1945; LaBenne and Greene, 1969; Maslow, 1954, 1970; Mead, 1934; Rogers, 1951; Stringer, 1971).

1. Personal adequacy is a universal basic need. Self-enhancement, self-fulfillment, self-actualization, and self-realization are fundamental drives, common to all. "Personal worth is not something human beings are free to take or leave. We must have it and when it is unattainable, everybody suffers" (Dobson, 1974, p. 13).

2. An individual's mental health and personal adjustment depend deeply on his sense of personal adequacy.

3. People behave in ways that are consistent or congruent with their self-concept. "A person's self is known to be the immediate determiner of his overt behavior" (Jourard, 1959, pp. 505-506).

4. A child's basic personality structure is established early in life and remains relatively stable over time.

5. The self abstraction is formed "in social intercourse, private reactions to himself, mastery in solving developmental tasks, and competence in dealing with life's situations" (Coopersmith, 1967, p. 20).

6. Although there is a tendency toward a unified global self, one's self-concept can be multidimensional with many referent groups (identifiable and distinct groups with which one associates).

7. Until threatened with exposure, an individual can tolerate a certain amount of inconsistency in self-concept and behavior from one situation to another and from one referent group to another.

8. One's self-concept is reinforced or modified by every life experience, especially those occurring during the maturing years. Its development continues throughout life either by conscious choice or incidentally by unconscious accident.

9. An individual's self-esteem determines how he interprets the perceptions from his social and physical environment.

10. An individual's self-esteem is determined by the interpretations given to the perceptions from his social and physical environment.
11. Self-esteem results from satisfaction of the basic need to value self and to be valued by others.
12. "The love for my own self is inseparably connected with the love for any other self. ... The attitudes towards others and towards ourselves, far from being contradictory, are basically conjunctive" (Fromm, 1947, p. 129).
13. Self-esteem, rather than being fixed, is responsive to changes in time, space, situational demands, and many other factors.
14. Threats to the self-concept or perceived inconsistencies between experience and self-concept may alter one's level of self-esteem.
15. "Satisfaction of the self esteem need leads to feelings of self-confidence, worth, strength, capability, and adequacy, of being useful and necessary in the world. But thwarting of these needs produces feelings of inferiority, of weakness, of helplessness" (Maslow, 1970, p. 45).

As abstract constructs, self-concept and self-esteem are subject to measurement difficulties. Fitts (1967), the author of the Tennessee Self-Concept Scale, suggested that "self description can be studied, analyzed, and scored in terms of such dimensions as: (1) the certainty or clarity of the image, (2) the defensiveness or distortion in the image, (3) the positive or negative flavor of the image, (4) the confusion and contradiction of the image" (p. 1). The precision of measurement is determined by the following factors as summarized by Combs (1963): "1. the clarity of the individual's awareness, 2. availability of adequate symbols of expression, 3. the willingness of the individual to cooperate, 4. the social expectancies, 5. the individual feeling of personal adequacy, 6. his feelings of freedom from threats" (p. 494). As imprecise as the current measures are, they are still a potential indicator of how a person perceives himself, (what he is, ought to be, or would like to be) and how he feels about himself, as long as they are used with caution.

SELF-ESTEEM AND REFLECTIONS

Discovery of the Physical Self

The formation of the self-concept begins in infancy and continues throughout life. The physical self is the first component of the self-concept to emerge in infancy. Most children use their vision to observe their own body and bodily actions as well as the objects, people, and actions within their social and physical environment. As a result, they normally begin to realize they are unique, distinct, and separate from that which is "not me." Later the child learns to place value judgments on the "good me" and the "bad me" (Sullivan. 1953).

Although the sequence of growth and development is essentially the same for the blind and the sighted, some of the developmental tasks are learned more slowly or at a later age by blind children (Fraiberg, 1977; Halliday, 1970; Lowenfeld, 1971). Awareness of the varied objects and persons both near and far, refinement of motor proficiency, locomotion, hand-ear coordination, bonding between mother and child, stimulation of exploration, and establishment of object and person permanence will develop in the blind child. However, adaptations or modifications may be required for maximum development.

> The concepts of person permanence and object permanence are essential for the development of a self-concept for three reasons. First, through person and object permanence, the baby learns to differentiate himself from his parents and from the surrounding environment. He begins unconsciously to comprehend that he is a separate being who can act on the world in which he lives. Second, after comprehending permanence, the infant will search for objects and persons because he knows they exist 'out there'; through his repeated experiences with those things or persons, he begins to learn that he can make things happen. Third, the infant then feels secure enough to release familiar objects or persons so that he can explore the environment further. It is through exploration and actions that the child discovers more completely his abilities and the strengths that contribute to a healthy self-concept. (Cook-Clampert, 1981, p. 236)

The process of differentiating oneself as a distinct and

autonomous being and the process of differentiating objects, animals, persons, or events from each other are more difficult for the congenitally blind child (Davis, 1964). In a longitudinal study of congenitally blind infants Fraiberg (1977) found delays in the establishment of a unique and distinct "I." However with intervention, "in those areas of development where comparative data are available, our educationally advantaged blind infants came closer to sighted-child ranges than blind-child ranges" (Fraiberg, 1977, p. 283).

Referring to a blind child's acquisition of a body image primarily through tactile and verbal means, Scholl (1973) concluded "these avenues are inferior in providing information concerning his body as compared to the bodies of others. Thus the formation of a body image is delayed" (p. 76). Cratty and Sams (1968) developed a body image test for blind children and found that, with systematic intervention, these lags could be remediated.

A good body image is the core of a healthy self-concept, while a poor body image can only result in a distorted self-concept. There is a direct correlation between feelings about one's body and feelings about the self (Secord and Jourard, 1953; Weinberg, 1960). When the body is physically impaired, as with blindness, the individual is frequently placed either by himself or by others in an inferior position, viewed as less competent and adequate. According to Adler (1950), this causes the individual to strive for superiority by maximizing special abilities as demonstrated for example in musical, athletic, or intellectual achievements. It should be noted that the inferior position is not inherent in blindness, but is frequently the status conferred on the blind person.

> But at the age of fourteen, through wrestling I wedged my foot in the door to the sighted world, the world that almost everyone else took for granted. My determination to barge my way through that door became brutal. Now I constantly searched about for ways to enter the world of the nonhandicapped.
>
> The next opportunity came about through music [after a voice test]. ... The maestro spun on his stool and said with high enthusiasm, "Tommy, you have a very fine voice indeed, and you have perfect pitch." If he had told me I'd just run the mile in three minutes or

inherited the crown of Ruritania I could not have been more elated. Here, anyway, was another field in which I could compete with sighted people on the basis of equality. (Sullivan and Gill, 1975, pp. 63-64)

The Reflected Self

An individual comes to know himself as he sees himself reflected in other people (Cooley, 1902). He attaches more importance to the reflections from the significant other, that is, "the people who most intimately administer the 'rewards' and 'punishments' in a person's life" (LaBenne and Greene, 1969, p. 14). Just as he learns to appreciate himself as he is appreciated by others, so too, he learns to devaluate himself as he is devaluated by others.

> The new school made me suddenly aware, as I never was before, of my blindness. It gave me an urgent need, a craving, for straight-forward, reliable feedback from the immediate environment. I wanted to be able to look into a mirror and say, "I look okay." I wanted to be able to check people's faces, their eyes, double-check that their reaction to something I said was what I thought it was. (Hartman and Asbell, 1978, pp. 58-59)

To illustrate this principle, a visually impaired person (VI) formulates opinions and judgments about his personal attributes (PA) primarily by the interaction with his social environment. The PA are the qualities and characteristics he believes to be true about himself. They include physical, mental, and emotional traits and abilities, characteristics of family and peer relations, values and attitudes, hopes and fears. The sum of the PA constitutes his perception of the self. The PA may be realistic or unrealistic; they may be firmly bonded or distorted and fragmented.

At the same time, each of the people who are significant to VI, such as a parent, teacher, or friend, has developed some notions about VI ("SO" will be used to refer to a significant other, representing any of the many significant others in VI's life.) These defining attributes (DA) are the characteristics and traits that SO ascribes to VI. As is true of the PA, the DA can range from very realistic to totally unrealistic. In Figure 4, the circle labeled VI represents the sum of all the

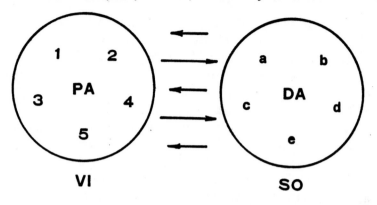

Figure 4. The Self and the Reflected Self

PA, his notions about himself (the self). The circle labeled SO is the sum total of all the DA, the notions SO assumes to be true about VI. A number is used to represent a PA and a letter to represent a DA. VI perceives SO's DA as reflections of himself and they formulate his reflected self.

Hartman found the reflections from his itinerant teacher to be positive, while Fries found some reflections from his peers to be negative.

> In short, Mrs. Landis taught me confidence—that a big, vague glob of emotional turmoil can be reduced to specifics; that something can be done about almost anything; that any person, even a blind person, can manage his environment enough to claim a guiding control over the course of his life. I came to believe that there is rarely an excuse for any person to feel like a helpless cork on a rolling sea, even though many people live all the days of their lives feeling that way. (Hartman and Asbell, 1978, p. 61)

> As I remember my boyhood a chief worry was my looks. Peers made fun of my straight blond hair, which Father cut bowl fashion. My glasses led to name calling of "Blindy", or "Four-eyes". I was convinced that I was the homeliest member of the family. This concerned me as I was sure no girl would ever be interested in a homely fellow like me. (Fries, 1980, p. 366)

The young, dependent, or immature VI, not trusting his own judgments about himself, tends to adopt the SO's judgments in preference to his own. The more dependent VI is, the more likely he is to accept without question SO's opinions regarding his attributes. "The abilities of the blind person are likely to continue to be underestimated by the public just because of its sighted vantage point" (Wright, 1974, p. 115). The persistent negative DA of the SO have a way of inevitably becoming VI's own PA, the basis of his self-concept and self-esteem.

Reflections that are approving produce feelings of self-approval. "In our society, almost everyone's self-esteem is strongly determined by the presence of approval or accept-ing-responses from others; but there is also great variability to be found in just how a person needs others to act toward him in order to maintain self-esteem" (Jourard, 1963, p. 145).

> It was a tired, hungry, happy blind athlete who sat at the dinner table that night. Larry [his brother] was as happy as I was. He had believed that blindness held no limitations for me, therefore it didn't. He felt that I could do everything that he was able to do, therefore I could.
>
> It was this confidence which I received from every member of my family that gave me the strength to attempt, to fail and to try again until the goal, whatever it happened to be, was achieved. (Krents, 1972, p. 102)

Sources of Personal Attributes and Defining Attributes

These PA and DA have their origin in a variety of experiences both at the conscious and unconscious levels. Because of the low incidence of blindness, the PA and DA are not easily validated or confirmed from a broad base of experience. The initial PA and DA, which may be based on the following sources, although potentially subject to later modification, color much of the early interaction between VI and SO.

1. Direct personal experience with other persons who are visually impaired (Bateman, 1962):

> I've forgotten her name now but I remember clearly how dark and musty her parlor was and how old she seemed. It turned out that she had graduated from Perkins only a year or two before, but to me she seemed a parchment person of greatly advanced age. Instantly I wondered if I would become like that if I went to her school. This poor woman probably gave such an impression only because she was totally inactive, completely isolated from the mainstream of life, which was

the case with most blind people, especially women at that time. (Caulfield, 1960, pp. 9-10)

2. Commonly held public attitudes and expectations about blindness (see Chapter 3):

I hadn't liked the excessively solicitous care received at the hotel nor the general air of hushed reverence with which it was offered. But this complete avoidance of the subject by my friend I liked no better. Then what the devil did I want. People were merely trying to be kind, helpful. Even if I could decide what I wanted, can a man have the nerve to tell the world in just what way he wants it to be kind?

I put the question up to my friend. He considered it carefully. "What you don't seem to have taken into your calculations," he said, "is the idea that you will be expected to conform."

"Conform to what?" I asked.

"To a type. You're the blind man now, you'll be expected to act like one."

"I don't want to be a type," I said.

"I don't say that you had to be one, I said you'd be expected to act like one. Everybody is expected to act his type if he doesn't want trouble." (Chevigny, 1946, p. 71)

3. The media portrayals of blind persons through television, movies, newspapers, and magazines:

If the media emphasizes the succumbing aspects of blindness, then the primary emotion aroused is derogatory pity. If, on the other hand, they emphasize the coping aspects of blindness, then the primary emotion elicited is respect and admiration (Wright, 1960). The following headlines typify the variety of factual and emotional styles of journalism.

"Although Blind, He Achieves Much" (*Greeley Tribune*, Nov. 26, 1975, p. 26)

"Reading Machine for Blind Promises New Freedoms" (*Denver Post*, Jan. 22, 1978, p. 41)

"Blind Man Sees Benefits to Building Own House" (*Sacramento Bee*, May 23, 1978)

Chevigney, a journalist himself, made an effort to prevent journalism that emphasized the succumbing aspects of blindness.

Sometime after I had returned to work, a New York newspaper

columnist indicated her desire to do a feature story on me. An invitation came in a roundabout way, through my agents. Nor did I see her when it came time to do the interviewing. She had what we call in the business a leg man talk to me. I didn't catch on to her real reason at first; columnists are busy people, most of them have assistants, and after all I wasn't Humphrey Bogart. Only later on, after the story appeared in print, did I learn that she couldn't bear to meet me because, as it was explained to me, she just knew she'd burst into tears. Together the leg man and I worked out a humorous piece, and the copy which I approved for publication had that feeling to it. The columnist who had never met me, however, just couldn't see it that way and rewrote the whole thing, the tears she hadn't shed on meeting me now falling into the typewriter. When she got through I was firmly endowed with all those characteristics, such as grit, stamina, and courage, which make most third-grade pupils look with such a jaundiced eye on literary heroes. It was all so tragic and I was being so brave. It was awful pretty, though, as a piece of writing—too bad it made my next two appointments so difficult to get. (Chevigny, 1946, p. 138)

4. The "attribution" and "spread" phenomenon:

Attribution is the process of attributing all of one's problems to blindness (Wright, 1974). For example, an individual may believe that because a person is blind, he is also helpless and dependent. Through spread, "the person is seen as disabled not only with respect to physique but with respect to other characteristics as well" (Wright, 1960, p. 71). For example an individual, observing a blind person having difficulty expressing himself, concludes that the speech disorder is caused by blindness.

I found, with some people, that as soon as they realized that I was blind, a subtle change had taken place in their attitude towards me. I had now become one of THE BLIND, incapable of moving about safely and in constant need of care and protection. I resentfully imagined that they thought that with the loss of sight had come loss of the ability to think for myself. (Hickford, 1973, p. 20-21)

5. Continued overt or subtle discrimination against per-persons who are visually impaired:

There are administrators of rehabilitation agencies and schools for the blind who philosophize about capable, independent blind persons, but who seem reluctant

to employ qualified visually impaired staff.
6. The manner in which VI presents himself:
   "Self-presentation may convince a person for the moment that he is indeed what he says he is" (Gergan, 1971, p. 86). Self-presentation can also convince others and will determine how he is perceived by them, thus influencing their defining attributes of VI.

> Most people relate only to the disability whatever the disability, but not to the individual. Part of the responsibility for that is society's but part is also the responsibility of the person who has the disability. If I constantly see myself as an incompetent, unable individual who is less than anyone else, that's going to be conveyed and other individuals are going to respond either by withdrawal, by pity or by overreacting. However, if I convey confidence, even if I fumble, even if I trip, even if I fall, it makes a difference. It's in the way that you feel about yourself. We all interrelate with each other. We all react to each other. (Sperber, 1976, pp. 230-231)

7. VI's aspiration and goals:
   Personal attributes and defining attributes may be ascribed to VI simply on the basis of what he wishes to become (Gergan, 1971). For example, if a person wishes to become a minister or priest, certain attributes or traits are immediately imputed to him.
   The initial attributes that are identified from these sources are often unrealistically positive or negative. Fortunately, they are subject to modification based upon subsequent interaction between VI and SO; usually this results in the reformulation of attributes that are more realistic.

Refining the Reflected Self

Some of the personal attributes and defining attributes may be in harmony with each other while others may be contradictory and dissonant. The visually impaired person and the significant other may share some common opinions about VI's characteristics and traits and they may totally disagree on others. The extent of the agreement between the PA and DA is, in large measure, a determiner of the extent of harmony in that relationship. Incompatibility tends to produce friction, dissonance, discord. When the respective attributes are at the level of awareness, shared PA and DA reinforce, while unshared threaten.

In Figure 5 the circles on the left illustrate how two individuals may share only two attributes, "2b" and "7g," which could be physical characteristics of height and weight, while disagreeing on all others, creating a climate for discord. The circles on the right represent two individuals who share many common judgments of the attributes of VI, and this is apt to result in a more harmonious relationship.

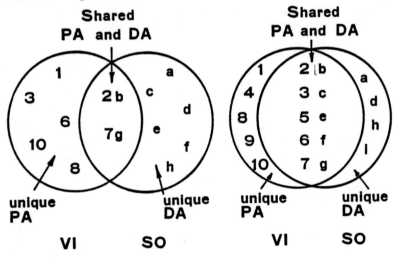

Figure 5. Quality of Relationship Determined by Extent of Shared Attributes

Krents described a situation in which his PA and the other's DA had little in common, thus producing conflict.

"Please forget everything I've said. I had no idea that you were er—ah—er"

"Blind," I volunteered.

"I'm not going to be able to sleep all night."

"Don't concern yourself about it," I said.

"You know," he confided, "my grandson is afflicted, too."

"Really?" I said.

"Yes. He's mentally retarded."
For a moment I stood there trying to control myself. Such comments tend to make me bitter. (Krents, 1972, p. 16)

Most people do not enjoy incompatible or discordant relationships. There is a natural striving to reduce friction by eliminating or circumventing any disagreements between PA and DA. Thus, reduction of dissonance can be accomplished by modifying VI's personal attributes or SO's defining attributes or, more likely, both in order to bring the DA and PA more in line with each other (to be discussed further in Chapter 6).

Young children still in their formative years, teen-agers in their struggle for identity, and immature, dependent adults are all susceptible to the defining attributes of their significant others. Because their personal attributes are not well established, they are more likely to abandon their own PA and adopt the corresponding incompatible DA as their own. In this way, they learn to define themselves more in terms of the defining attributes of others.

Figure 6 illustrates how VI abandons his own personal

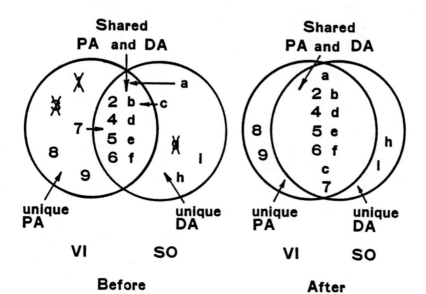

Figure 6. Adopting Discrepant Defining Attributes

attributes "1" and "3" in favor of SO's defining attributes "a" and "c." At the same time SO alters his opinion of attribute "g" to be more in keeping with VI's opinion represented by "7." The process results in an increased number of shared attributes.

The following excerpt illustrates how significant others altered their defining attributes in favor of Mitchell's personal attributes.

> Soon after I learnt that my failing sight would ultimately lead to blindness, I passed on the information by letter to two old and true friends. In each case I had by letter a warm and sympathetic response, but in each case when next I came in personal contact with these friends, I sensed at once a nervous reaction, a doubt as to what changes they would find in me and what was the right way to behave. Luckily I did sense this nervousness and set about combating it by being as natural and normal as I could, a course which was successful, bringing my relationship with these two friends quickly back on its old easy footing. It was a useful experience, teaching me right at the beginning that besides learning to take blindness in my stride, I had to persuade my friends to take it in theirs. (Mitchell, 1964, p. 87)

Definition and redefinition of the self continues throughout life by means of the reflected appraisals (Sullivan, 1953). VI's personal attributes are reinforced when he encounters DA that match his PA. When there is disagreement, then VI must evaluate the appraisor and the appraisal to determine whether to accept or reject the discrepant defining attribute (Gergan, 1971). If the appraisor is judged to be credible, or appears to be warm and caring, then his defining attributes are more readily accepted. The more positive, the more frequent, and the more consistent the confirming appraisals are, the more apt they are to modify or replace existing personal attributes.

The Reflected Self and the Physical Environment

In addition to VI's personal attributes and SO's defining attributes, the context or physical environment contributes to the quality of the interaction. Situational demands or distractions may make the visually impaired person uncomfortable, and this discomfort may be erroneously interpreted by others as disinterest or unfriendliness. The newly blinded tend to be preoccupied when practicing a recently acquired adaptive skill. Attention will continue to be diverted away from social interaction until that skill becomes routine and automatic.

> One of my first reactions to blindness was to refuse any invitation which included a meal, even at the home of friends. I didn't want to apper conspicuous and resented having my food cut for me. This problem was solved with my first meal at the school [Seeing Eye]. (Clifton, 1963, p. 68)

When a person is not in customary control of himself within his environment, his anxiety level increases, putting a strain on his relationships with others. A blind person at a crowded party may find it quite difficult to mix freely with the guests, or to find a special friend. In a noisy setting the usual auditory clues may be masked, making a normally routine task difficult or impossible. In a strange or unfamiliar setting, his mental energies are absorbed in solving new problems and familiarizing himself in a new setting, drawing attention away from normal social intercourse.

> There was music in the background and a hubbub of voices; there was much laughter too and everyone seemed to be enjoying themselves hugely, but I found all the noises bewildering as I was unable to distinguish any individual voice and was completely unaware of anything that was said. There were, of course, people sitting on either side of me, but if either of them had spoken I had not heard a word. As I had already found out for myself since becoming blind, some people do not know how to approach a blind person and are often seemingly tongue-tied, so I knew that I must start a conversation myself. This I tried, but so far as I know, I received no reply; perhaps the answers were lost in the general hubbub. This tea party was going to be a nightmare, I thought: why was I there? (Hickford, 1977, p. 30)

The higher the level of preoccupation with solving the problems that the new situation demands, or the higher the level of anxiety over anticipating the new and different, the more ineffective VI becomes in his social interactions. His reduced effectiveness has two potential consequences: (1) SO may misunderstand and, perceiving social distance, may himself withdraw or may become oversolitous, and (2) VI may allow the temporary, situational reduced effectiveness to be generalized to a lowered self-esteem. The environmental setting illustrated in Figure 7 provides VI with a number of distractions that serve to divert his attention away from a bewildered SO.

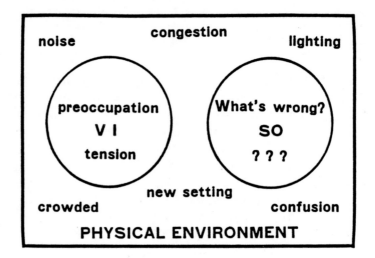

Figure 7. Situational Demands and Distractions

To a certain extent, everyone selects the situation and the setting that offer the greatest opportunity for self-enhancement, for maintaining a congenial self-concept (Hamachek, 1971). A witty person may choose to go to a party rather than a lecture, a blind person may choose a less noisy, less crowded, or more familiar setting when choice permits.

Reciprocal Reflections

While the visually impaired person is establishing his personal attributes with the help of the significant other's defining attributes, another process is occurring simultaneously. VI is concurrently developing some defining attributes of SO, certain attributes the blind person believes to be true about SO. At the same time, SO has a set of personal attributes he believes to be true about himself.

VI's defining attributes of SO are formulated from the same set of values and attitudes from which his own personal attributes were formulated. He tends to look for and selectively to perceive the attributes that are important to him.

A self-accepting person will be more accepting of others and will, in turn be more accepted by others. By the same token, a self-rejecting person will tend to reject others and be rejected by others (Hamachek, 1971). Being rejected by others reinforces his self-rejecting attitudes. A person with high self-esteem, by influencing the self-esteem of another, can reinforce his own high self-esteem.

Just as some sighted individuals have stereotypic attitudes that color their defining attributes of VI, some blind persons have stereotypic attitudes about the sighted that color their defining attributes of SO. They may become persuaded that all sighted are dominating tyrants, pitying patronizers, or fearful avoiders. These unhealthy and unjust stereotypic notions are just as damaging to the development of realistic PA and DA as are the negative attitudes toward the blind.

Multiple Significant Others

The analysis of the dynamics involved in the formulation of one's self-concept and self-esteem now becomes even more complex when one considers the multiple significant others. The reflective and reciprocal processes just described are repeated every time VI interacts with another SO, resulting in multiple social selves (James, 1890; Mead, 1934). Furthermore, not all the significant others share the same defining attributes of VI. Dad, sister, teacher, and friend may perceive and evaluate VI's attributes in different ways. The parent and school administrator in the following excerpt do not share the same defining attribute of Krents.

"When am I going back to school?" I asked her breathlessly.
I was ecstatic. I raced up the stairs and came sliding down the banister.
"I'm afraid that you can only go in the afternoons for a while," Mother said quietly.

I dropped to the floor with a thud and let my joy ooze out of me.
"I'm still different," I muttered. "You promised that once I could do long division, I could be just like all the others kids."
"Dr. Stover [the school administrator] still doesn't believe you're as smart as the other children." (Krents, 1972, p. 113)

The interaction between VI and the multiple others with a variety of environmental settings is portrayed in Figure 8.

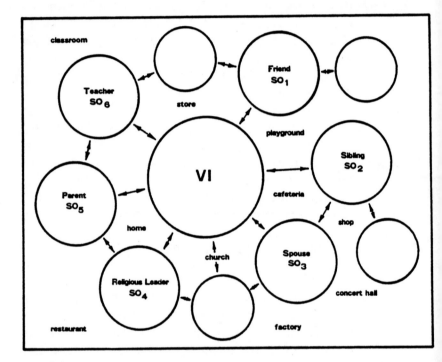

Figure 8. Multiple Significant Others, Acquaintances, and Environments

Each SO usually represents a referent group: family, church, classmates, gang, employees. The evaluative significance of certain traits or characteristics may vary from one referent group to another (Gergan, 1971). One group might attach great significance to academic abilities, another to brute strength, and yet another to economic independence. The overlapping roles prescribed by group membership may be compatible (son and student), interfering (residential school student and public school student), antagonistic (Baptist and atheist), or exluding (blind and pilot) (Meyerson, 1971).

VI's assimilation into a referent group depends on two factors: (1) VI's ability to play the role defined by the group and (2) the extent to which members of the referent group perceive the differences between their own personal attributes and their defining attributes of VI as significant. One's need for a sense of identity and sense of belonging is met by being assimilated into one or more of the referent groups.

> My social insecurities in college were not just with girls, of course. The reason I joined Sigma Chi was to advance the cause of feeling accepted. Once joining the fraternity, however, I encountered the old story of not only feeling uncomfortable until I felt accepted, but realizing that others were uncomfortable with me until they knew how to deal with me. I resorted to making jokes about my blindness. Jokes were very effective in relaxing people. They also gained attention, which I apparently crave, even though after gaining it I'd fret over whether I got it for the wrong reasons. . . .
>
> Inevitably, I realized that my little jokes, while at first relaxing people, eventually fixated them on me as a blind person, not as Dave Hartman. So I resolved to move away from snappy one-liners during tense social moments, but I didn't always succeed. To this day I reflexively reach for them. (Hartman and Asbell, 1978, pp. 105-106)

Nonassimilation or rejection by a referent group leads to feelings of worthlessness and lowered self-esteem.

> "Won't the kids be surprised tomorrow," I said to Mother as I climbed happily into bed. "Maybe they'll like me more now that I can see like they can. At last, I'm not different." . . .
> "What funny glasses," said one of my classmates.
> "Hey, you look like the Man from Mars," shouted another.
> My great surprise was ruined. My happiness lay in ashes all around me. I was still different; I was still lonely. . . .
> I sat in that classroom, hating the other children, hating the new glasses, and, most of all, hating myself for being blind. (Krents, 1972, p. 77)

Group members are expected to participate in group activities, to contribute to the group welfare, and to share in the group benefits. Persons who are visually impaired cannot, at one and the same time, expect both equal treatment and special concessions (Bauman and Yoder, 1962). Special provisions for the blind such as free mailing privileges, an extra income tax exemption, reduced rates on public transportation, although intended to facilitate assimilation, probably do more to perpetuate negative stereotypes and segregation, ostracizing the blind from the group called society.

SELF-ESTEEM AND RELATIONSHIPS

Some acquaintances become significant others, while some remain casual acquaintances. The greater the significance of the other, the greater the potency for influencing VI's personal attributes and self-esteem. There is a positive correlation between VI's level of self-esteem and the degree of warmth, care, and acceptance exhibited by SO (Coopersmith, 1967). Frequent and consistent encounters with even the casual acquaintance can also influence VI's self-concept. The young or immature visually impaired and the recently blinded are more vulnerable to, and less capable of evaluating, the perceived DA of even casual acquaintances.

Fitts (1970) discussed some underlying assumptions that govern interpersonal relationships. He believed that relationships are a universal need, and that communication at both the cognitive and affective levels is essential to good interpersonal relationships. The development of interpersonal relationships is a learned behavior that is facilitated by feedback. He maintained that the key assumption is "the behaviors and feelings involved in interpersonal relationships are subject to varying degrees of control by the individual" (p. 12).

Since both the type and the quality of relationships contribute to the nature and potency of the perceived defining attributes projected by the acquaintance, it would be helpful to analyze the effect of each on VI's self-esteem. Although the types described are not sequential in the sense that a person moves from one level to the next, each succeeding type demonstrates an improvement in the quality of the relationship.

The Non-person or Impersonal Relationship
The "It"

Some sighted acquaintances occasionally speak of the person who is visually impaired as though he were an object, referring to him as "it." Others converse about VI as if he were not present, totally ignoring him and excluding him from conversation. The direction of the effect on VI's self-esteem is obvious. The demeaning and devaluating relationship can only result in lowered self-esteem. In an effort to prove that he was more than an "it," Morgan resorted to stealing a record from a music store.

> "I'm frustrated by people, Mom. When people meet George [his brother] they see a neat guy who plays football and has girlfriends. When they meet me they don't even see a person. They see a pair of eyes that can't see them. That makes me less than a whole person to them. I think it's an ego thing. Because I can't see them I'm not worthy of their time. There isn't a day that I don't get turned off by people. It's like it was in grammar school. I'm blind so I must be retarded or spastic."
>
> "That's because of their own lack of knowledge, Dan. It's up to you to prove them wrong." .
>
> "I know. That's just what I tried today. It was like I was yelling, 'Look! A blind person can steal.'" (Morgan, 1979, p. 158)

The Relationship Based on Stereotypes
"The Blind"

Some individuals relate to a person who is visually impaired on the basis of common stereotypes: helpless, dependent, beggars, musical, having a sixth sense, using sign language, living in darkness, associated with sin. These stereotypes predispose the acquaintance to certain attitudes, which are reflected in the DA he projects. They expect VI to conform to a predetermined mold that is groundless and senseless. The impact on VI's self-concept and self-esteem is confining and degrading. Though Clifton was eighteen years old, some acquaintances believed that she was totally dependent, unable to care for herself.

> Some of our friends were aghast when they learned that Mother was going out to work. Wasn't she afraid to leave me alone? Wasn't she afraid I might hurt myself? One even sympathized with her because she would have to get up early so she could wash and dress me before going to work. (Clifton, 1963, p. 41)

The Relationship Based on the Exception "The Superblind"

Some acquaintances holding stereotypic notions of all blind people find it difficult to adjust their DA when encountering a well-adjusted, capable VI. Rather than adjusting their DA, they explain the apparent discrepancy by imputing super or exceptional qualities to VI. "He is the exception that proves the rule," they reason.

When VI is considerd remarkable and unusual for performing very ordinary and routine tasks, such as eating, telling time, telephoning, it has one of two possible consequences: (1) VI's self-esteem is unrealistically inflated or (2) VI recognizes the facade as masking the more generalized demeaning and devaluating attitude toward blindness.

> There is no denying that their flattering comments can be appealing, and that is the way to regard them rather than to remember what they are really implying by their high praise. . . . In other words all that their comments mean is best translated into "being blind, I suppose you have to fall back on other people for everything. But not you! You can do a few things on your own. You really are remarkable!" (Edwards, 1962, p. 35)

The Relationship Based on Succumbing "The Needy Blind"

A relationship based on the succumbing, dependent aspects of blindness serves to enhance the self-esteem of the acquaintance at the expense of VI's self-esteem. The acquaintance has a condescending, patronizing, oversolitous attitude, expecting VI to be indebted and grateful for all "acts of kindness and mercy." The root of this relationship is pity, and pity strips the recipient of personal integrity and worth.

My resistance started very young to the do-gooders who would call in to "take him out."

One of these, certainly the one I did more to dodge than anyone else, was a worthy, elderly woman, whom I shall call Miss Prudence. She worked as a superior help in various well-to-do houses. Every so often when she had a day off she would make it a day out for me too. I had to contend with her from the time I was seven until I was about fourteen when I refused to put up with any more of it. At intervals, which I did all I could to widen, she would call for me at the Blind School, or at home, and off we would go walking through parks and gardens around Melbourne or visiting some of her friends. . . .

If I had not been blind, I would not have had such attention. Certainly my brothers had no Miss Prudence to contend with. (Edwards, 1962, p. 46)

The Relationship Based on Coping "The Capable Blind"

In this relationship, the acquaintance recognizes that VI can become fairly independent by learning some basic skills and adaptive techniques and is devoted to fostering that independence. The recognition that he is capable, the expectation of performance, the development of coping skills, all have a positive influence on VI's self-esteem.

There was no one to show her how to cope with my training. Yet she [his mother] instinctively understood the importance of teaching me how to dress myself and how to feed myself without spilling food or knocking over cups.

She showed me, for instance, that I could avoid putting on a shirt inside out by feeling for the manufacturer's tag inside the collar. She devised a way for me to eat by using a piece of bread in my left hand as a pusher to the fork.

When I was quite young she helped me avoid the habits that make so many blind people awkward, embarrassing and unattractive. (Sullivan and Gill, 1975, p. 28)

The Relationship Based on Respect "The Person Who Is Blind"

The focus of this relationship is on respect and understanding for the individual person with all of his needs and desires, with all of his interests and capabilities, with all of his joys and sorrows. The fact that he is visually impaired is only incidental to the relationship. This acquaintance, too, will desire to see VI become as independent as possible, but the relationship has a much broader base. Respect and admiration for the individual person who is blind can have a powerfully positive impact on VI's self-esteem.

> He didn't care about my not being able to see. He could play a trick on me just as quickly as he would play one on anybody. That wasn't so bad; it was all right really. No, It was pretty good. No! It was wonderful! Gee! It was the nicest thing anyone had ever done for me. (Russell, 1962, p. 79)

The Relationship Based on Friendship "The Friend Who Happens to Be Blind"

In this relationship, in addition to respect, the acquaintance develops an attraction for, an affection for the individual who, among many other qualities, happens to be blind. Friendship is a relationship of both giving and receiving, of mutual respect. As a result, VI's self-esteem is enhanced immeasurably with the knowledge that he contributes to someone else's welfare and happiness.

> For the first time since I could remember, I had a chance to make friends with sighted boys and girls my own age, who, after the initial awkwardness of my being blind, accepted me as one of them, ducking my head under water, pushing me off the low diving board, sometimes trying to make me lose my directions in the swimming pool. Ed, who always sat facing the pool and kept a watchful eye on the swimmers, at first used to scold them. "Don't you know any better," he used to say, "than to treat a blind person like that?" . . .
> I knew I had to make friends with Ed, to make him understand that I would rather be hurt in the swimming pool than be left alone. . . .
> He stopped, too, trying to protect me in the swimming pool, and whenever I did have a rough time, I sensed that he watched with a gleeful eye, and I was glad that I played chess with him ruthlessly. (Mehta, 1957, pp. 266-267)

A relationship based on friendship sometimes leads to marriage.

> The first twenty-five years of my life had been a long uphill struggle to function successfully in the sighted world. I had a family whose faith in God and confidence in me never faltered. Ours was a team effort which had made it possible for me to be in a position now where I could proudly ask Kit to share a very full and exciting life with me. . . .

But as Kit squeezed my hand, I knew that as far as she was concerned, none of these things made any difference. I was simply the man with whom she was in love. We were a man and woman, eagerly looking forward to spending a lifetime together. Nothing else mattered, least of all my blindness. (Krents, 1972, p. 12)

Both the acquaintance and the visually impaired person share equally in the responsibility for the type of relationship established. If the acquaintance thrives on succumbing, then that's probably where their relationship will start. If VI views himself as a stereotype, then that too is probably where the relationship begins.

After a relationship begins to develop, it can stagnate at a particular level or it can mature into a warm, wholesome, mutually satisfying one. It should be of no concern if a relationship begins at the first four levels. The real concern is if, after a period of time, it remains at one of those levels.

Walt was the first blind person I had ever known well. Our relationship went through the several stages that I have come to know in relationships with others. At first I was simply astounded by the novelty of the way he lived.... As our relationship matured the novelty disappeared and he became a normal person to me. I paid him the compliment I desire now for myself: I forgot about his blindness. (Kemper, 1977, p. 122)

Although the captain's relationship with Caulfield began at the stereotypic level, it moved to a much stronger position.

"Well," the captain said apologetically, "I expected to see you come aboard in a wheel chair. I didn't think you would be able to take a step without somebody holding on to your arm. I certainly didn't expect to find you walking around the deck and going into the dining room by yourself. And the last thing I expected was that, instead of us helping you, you would end up helping us run the ship." (Caulfield, 1960, p. 74)

VI must remember that he carried the burden of the responsibility for putting the acquaintance at ease about blindness.

My task was to put the men I'd come to see at their ease—the reverse of the usual situation. Curiously, I found it much easier to do with men I'd never met before. Perhaps this was because with strangers there was no body of reminiscences to cover before business could be gotten down to and so there was no unpleasant contrast with the present. (Chevigny, 1946, p. 136)

Enduring relationships are more likely to develop when people relate to others with whom they agree. It has been said that friendships are choosing one's own propaganda. If VI relates only with persons whose DA agree with his own PA, then he is seldom challenged to reevaluate his self-concept (Hamachek, 1971).

SELF-ESTEEM AND SELF-APPRAISAL

As the child grows and matures and his powers of abstraction increase, he is better able to symbolize, evaluate, and integrate or reject those life's experiences that potentially bear upon self-esteem. With the increasing complexity of the self-abstraction, the process of reflected appraisals becomes more selective. "Selectivity results in certain attributes being excluded and others being overemphasized. The self—that is, the object a person regards himself to be—is selectively weighted according to the individual's abstraction of the common features of his personal experiences" (Coopersmith, 1967, p. 21).

Self-esteem emerges from VI's evaluation of his personal attributes, some of which are more significant than others in their contribution to VI's self-esteem. According to Wright (1960), the more potent attributes are (1) the ones that have a closer connection to the "essential me" and (2) the ones representing higher value priorities. Attributes take on greater potency as they move closer to the torso and face (eyes more potent than fingers). Personal characteristics (appearance) have higher potency than personal actions (playing a guitar). Attributes of being (to be creative) have greater potency than attributes of having (to have hair). Depending on one's value system, an attribute representing a high value (honesty) has more potency than a lower value (punctuality). If permitted, one's self-esteem can be dominated and exclusively determined by a particularly sensitive personal attribute such as blindness. In this case all other characteristics, traits, and abilities seem to dwindle into insignificance.

> Sometimes I feel that everything and anything I ever achieve will be linked inseparably to my blindness, the blindness being more important than the achievement—or the achiever. "Did you hear what that blind doctor's done now? Yeah, wow, blind!" Someday I'd like to do something totally independent of blindness, something that might be written about, without the writer saying that this guy can't see. I hope someday to accomplish that. (Hartman and Asbell, 1978, p. 26)

Part of the self-evaluation process is to be able to see oneself as others do. Blind persons, especially children, tend to find it more difficult to take another's place and to view themselves from the other's perspective. The tendency toward isolation, toward ego-centrism, and the lags in conceptualization discussed in Chapter 3 all contribute to this difficulty. The ability to evaluate oneself from another's frame of reference aids in discriminating valid from invalid reflected appraisals. When an individual understands the values and attributes that determine the significant other's DA of himself, then he is in a better position to understand, modify, accept, or reject SO's defining attributes and their evaluative loadings. This requires self-transcendence, the ability to rise above one's own private motives and thoughts in order better to understand and share another's perspective (Hamachek, 1971).

The significant other makes judgments about VI's esteem, worth, or value in a very similar manner. SO weights each DA by his own values and attitudes. Thus, the same attribute found among both PA and DA may contribute quite differently to estimations of VI's esteem or worth.

Just as attributes are learned by reflections from others, so are feelings of esteem and worth. VI comes to value himself as he is valued by others (Symonds, 1951). People tend to be attracted to those who evaluate them positively and dislike those who evaluate them negatively (Gergan, 1971). Through reflected appraisals, the self emerges as either disparaging and hostile or as positive and approving (Sullivan, 1953). "Generally, a high regard for one's self is reflected in a high level of personal adjustment" (Hamachek, 1971, p. 231).

SUMMARY

The process of developing self-esteem is the same for all persons whether blind or sighted. One comes to know himself as he sees himself reflected in others, particularly the significant others. He comes to feel about himself as he perceives that others feel toward him. Comparing a person's perception of himself with other's perceptions of him and resolving and circumventing basic differences is a process that is repeated with each new relationship. Interactions with social and physical environment, the types and qualities of those interactions, the perceived attributes and feelings of all parties concerned are essential ingredients in the development of one's self-concept and one's self-esteem. As such, this process is primarily externally oriented. In the next chapter, self-esteem as a product of the evaluation of one's competence is presented as a more internally oriented process.

Chapter 5.

SOURCES OF SELF-ESTEEM, INTERNALLY ORIENTED

There are two primary sources of self-esteem, external and internal. The last chapter described the externally oriented sources as reflections from others. The younger, the more immature, or the more dependent a person is, the more he relies on approval from others for his self-esteem. In fact, for some, seeking the approval of others has become a stronger drive than satisfying basic physiological needs (Rogers, 1951).

The second source of self-esteem is more internally oriented and becomes increasingly prominent as the person grows older, more mature, or more independent. As was mentioned in the last chapter, these sources of self-esteem are not unique to individuals who are visually impaired. They emerge from general psychological principles that operate in all persons, whether blind or sighted. "Self-esteem cannot thrive indefinitely on just the approval from other people. Sooner or later it has to be supported by proof of one's worth, by one's becoming competent, productive and responsible, and this proof of worth in turn feeds into one's interpersonal relationships and enriches them" (Stringer, 1971, p. 119).

The overview of blindness provided in Chapters 2 and 3 developed the theme that, all other things being equal, persons who are visually impaired are potentially capable of, but may lack the opportunity for, proving their competence. Since feelings of competence are a major source of self-esteem, and since their attainment is more difficult for persons who are visually impaired, professionals need to assist blind persons to develop and exercise competence, productivity, and responsibility.

Coopersmith's (1967) review of literature and exploratory research into the antecedents of self-esteem centered around four ingredients or conditions that contribute to self-esteem: successes, defenses, values, and aspirations. While defenses are not dealt with until Chapter 6 in this book, the other three factors are incorporated into the cyclical process described in this chapter.

One of the major sources of VI's self-esteem is the continuous internal process of making judgments about his own competence. Out of one's personal attributes emerge his aspirations and goals in life. A person's aspirations determine the tasks and activities he chooses to accomplish. His performance of these tasks and activities is evaluated against a standard of his own choosing. Judgments about the extent of success in accomplishing one's goals are weighted by the salience and significance of the value of that task or activity. Weighted judgments of success or failure have a tendency to either reinforce or modify one's estimates of his own personal attributes (including his self-esteem), which, in turn, determine future aspirations and goals. This cyclical process continuously makes an impact upon a visually impaired person's feeling of competence and adequacy.

While this internally oriented process is occurring within the visually impaired individual, a similar process is operating within the significant others, providing the basis for additional reflections. Out of the defining attributes SO establishes certain expectations, observes VI's performance, judges success by SO's own standards, and weights the significance of the success by his own value system. This process serves as a basis for reinforcing or modifying SO's defining attributes of VI. With the newly strengthened or revised defining attributes, the cycle begins once more.

These two cyclical processes for VI and SO are occurring simultaneously. Each step of VI's process can affect and be affected by its counterpart in SO's process in the reflective manner described in Chapter 4, providing many opportunities for discrepancies and conflicts to occur. Figure 9 illustrates VI's cycle and SO's cycle occurring at the same

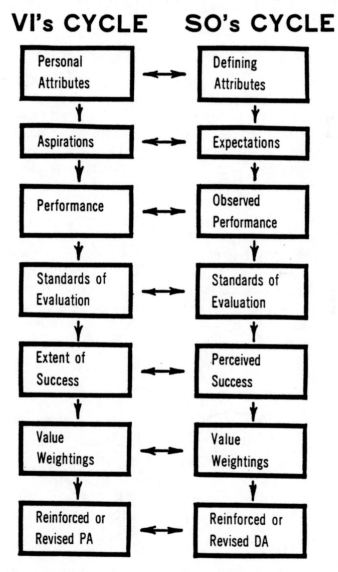

VI's CYCLE   SO's CYCLE

VI's CYCLE	SO's CYCLE
Personal Attributes	Defining Attributes
Aspirations	Expectations
Performance	Observed Performance
Standards of Evaluation	Standards of Evaluation
Extent of Success	Perceived Success
Value Weightings	Value Weightings
Reinforced or Revised PA	Reinforced or Revised DA

Figure 9. Sources of VI's Self-esteem—The Internal Process Interacting with the External Process

time, with the possibility of interaction between the two at every step.

The remainder of this chapter analyzes these two cycles in more detail. Due to their simultaneous nature, it seems best to discuss the two processes concurrently, one step at a time.

VI'S ASPIRATIONS AND SO'S EXPECTATIONS

The visually impaired person's aspirations and self-expectations are rooted in his estimates of his own personal attributes. Aspirations refer to one's long- and short-range goals and objectives. Self-expectations refer more to VI's prediction of his own behavior in response to specific stimuli. At the same time, the significant others have expectations of VI that include both future goals and predicted responses.

In Figure 10, SO_2 and SO_3 could represent father and mother who share some but not all expectations of VI (symbolized by letters). Some of the father's expectations coincide with some but not all of VI's aspirations (symbolized by numbers) and the same is true for mother's expectations. SO_1 could represent a friend who does not share any expectations with father and mother, but some of his expectations do coincide with some of VI's aspirations.

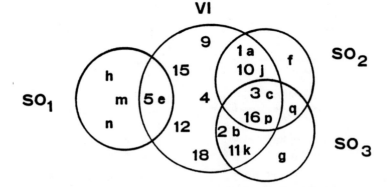

Figure 10. VI's Aspirations and SO's Expectations, Shared and Unshared

Finally each has expectations or aspirations that are shared by no one else.

Obviously, VI's aspirations and self-expectations are not shared by all significant others. Neither does VI share all expectations of the significant others. Furthermore, the significant others do not all share common expectations of VI. The unshared aspirations and expectations are potential sources of friction and conflict.

VI's Aspirations

Aspirations are based on an individual's estimate of his capacities to meet the demands of the chosen tasks and activities. Depending on the feedback from the social and physical environment, VI's estimates of his capacities can vary from moment to moment, from person to person, and from situation to situation. They can also vary from unrealistically high to unrealistically low, which of course includes the possibility that they are realistic. As a general rule "people aspire to do that which will yield success and shun activities which may lead to failure" (Gergan, 1971, p. 77).

> Bill had light perception but no useful vision. When I asked him one Friday afternoon to tighten a set of damper flange screws before making repairs, he surprised me by saying, "The blind can't do that."
> "Where did you get that idea?" I rejoined.
> "Mr. Dry [former teacher who was sighted] never said it but he might as well have. Every time when Mr. Dry worked on dampers he said, 'I need to focus the light into the action to spot the right screw without dislodging a spring or two.' If he couldn't put the right screw by touch, why expect me to do it?" (Fries, 1980, p. 220)

People usually set goals that are attainable, or nearly so. In a study comparing aspiration level of blind and sighted ten to fifteen year olds, McAndrew (1948) found no significant difference when the subjects were asked how firmly they could squeeze a hand dynamometer. Coopersmith (1967) found that high self-esteem children set higher goals for themselves than did low self-esteem children and they came closer to reaching those higher goals. He further reported that among the high self-esteem children there is a higher level of confidence in their own abilities to achieve their goals. "Accomplishment of a personal goal, whether in a physical, or intellectual, or social realm, can be a self-enhancing experience to the extent that it is personally meaningful and not too easily won" (Hamachek, 1971, p. 243).

SO's Expectations

The significant others' expectations of VI are based on their estimations of VI's capacities. When these expectations are realistic, they can serve to encourage and motivate the visually impaired person on to greater and greater accomplishments. The expectations of parents of high self-esteem children instill confidence in their children (Coopersmith, 1967). Whether realistic or not, expectations play a powerful role in shaping the behavior of others for "people more often than not do what is expected of them, and they become what they are thought to be" (LaBenne and Greene, 1969, p. 43). "When the adults in a child's life demonstrate that they firmly believe a skill may be mastered, the child will begin to convince herself. Constant encouragement and praise of work well done will help a child maintain the persistence required for eventual mastery" (Mangold, 1982, p. 98).

> [Mama] never let me get away with anything just 'cause I was blind. I was treated like I was normal. I acted like I was normal. And I wound up doing exactly the same things normal people do. (Charles and Ritz, 1978, p. 43)

After studying role expectations and performance of blind children, Mayadas (1972) concluded that "role synchrony existed between performance of blind subjects and (1) expectations of significant others, (2) subject's perception of significant other expectations and (3) subject's self-expectations. Role asynchrony was indicated between expectations of persons who were strangers to the blind and the role performance of blind subjects" (p. 48).

The expectations of others are a prime molder of VI's own view of independence. The more dependent VI is, the more he will attempt to comply with the expectations of others. The more independent he is, the more he is likely to defy or withstand others' expectations for dependency (Lukoff and Whiteman, 1970).

Expectations of VI that are too low are frequently ground-ed in the devaluating negative attitudes discussed in Chapter 3. For example, others expected Hocken to be a liability solely on the basis of her blindness.

> But finding a flat wasn't so easy. The difficulties arose not because of a shortage of accommodation, but mainly because I was blind. So many times we turned up for an appointment, and as Anita told me afterwards, the face of the prospective landlord or landlady dropped when he or she realized I could not see. What kind of liability, I wonder, did they expect me to be? Would I blunder around and smash the furniture, overflow the bath and bring the plaster down, or simply cause the entire house to go up in flames? (Hocken, 1977, pp. 72-73)

Unrealistically low expectations manifest themselves when the significant other attempts to overprotect, dominate, or patronize the person who is blind. When VI attempts to meet these low expectations, he succeeds at less than his optimum, resulting in the potential for either lowered self-esteem or inflated self-esteem. On the other hand the more independent blind individual, upon encountering low expectations as Dahl did, will continue to pursue his own goals.

> At the University of Minnesota, the dean of the College of Education had told me that I could never become a teacher; the students would know about my affliction and poke fun at me. (Dahl, 1962, p. 9)

Expectations that are unrealistically high can be equally damaging to VI's self-esteem.

> In contrast to overprotective parents are those who try to push the child to prove that he is "normal" and the same as (or better than) his sighted peers. Constant pressure to compete and succeed is damaging to any child. Under these conditions some children do not even try because they are afraid to fail. Those who try and fail to fulfill the expectations of significant others can easily come to view themselves as inadequate and worthless. (Cook-Clampert, 1981, p. 237)

Although Cook-Clampert was referring specifically to visually impaired children, the same thing could be said of a blind person of any age and his significant other.

> My mother didn't mind my going to work. She didn't like the idea of my working on a sewing machine, but she liked the idea of my getting out with people. My father objected.
> "I can support her," he said. "What will people think if I send my blind daughter out to work!" (Sperber, 1976, p. 81)

In addition to the conflict that arises from incompatible or unshared aspirations and expectations, there are other inconsistencies and contradictions that product confusion and/or friction. Sometimes a blind person's expectations of the sighted are themselves contradictory: "Treat me just like you treat anybody else" along with "I expect special provisions and concessions because I am blind." VI's aspirations themselves may also be contradictory: "I want to be independent and stand on my own two feet" and "I want to be dependent because I don't like the hassels of arguing with others." SO's expectations of VI can be contradictory: "I expect you to use braille, white cane, and other special techniques" and "I expect you to behave like a sighted person by looking at me when you talk to me and by refraining from rocking." Thus, there emerge basic questions that plague every mature young adult, blind or sighted: "Do I want to be dependent or independent?" "Am I living my life to please myself or to please others?" The answer to these questions, of course, is "yes."

VI'S PERFORMANCE AND OBSERVED PERFORMANCE

The aspirations of VI and the expectations of others determine, to a large extent, the endeavors VI undertakes. Self-esteem is related to performance or, more precisely, to competence demonstrated in performance. To be a competent adult, Bower (1966) suggested that an individual must learn to love, to have enough to oneself to share with another; to work, to contribute to the welfare of another; and to play, to relax, recreate, and enjoy oneself in his physical and social surroundings.

A person's sense of competence, a major contributor to self-esteem, is "his perception of the probability that his actions will attain his goals" (Stotland and Canon, 1972, p. 447). One's actual competence is differentiated from one's sense of competence and is defined by Argyris (1965) as "an individual's ability to produce intended effects in such a way that he can continue to do so" (p. 4). He suggested that the higher the level of competence the greater the awareness of actual and potential problems, the greater the ability to solve these problems, and the greater the ability to retain these skills into the future.

VI's Performance

VI's activities are not all designed to help him reach his goals. Many of them are undertaken to meet the expectations of others: parents, employers, teachers, and peers. Still others are simply responses to environmental stimuli (e.g. door-to-door salesmen) that may have nothing to do with either aspirations or expectations.

VI's sense of competence stems from his ability to detect or anticipate the demands to be made upon himself, to choose a course of action from several alternatives, and to solve problems that may arise. The perceived effectiveness of one's actions and thus a sense of competence is conditional on two factors: (1) an individual's having available many alternative courses of action from which to select the most effective way to reach his goal and (2) an individual's having a good understanding of the rules that govern a situation (Stotland and Canon, 1972). From earlier discussion, it is evident that, without compensatory behaviors, persons who are blind have less information upon which to build schemas and upon which to base decisions about alternative courses of action.

> Because I am blind, I run into all kinds of personal problems on which I feel bound to bow to the opinions of others. I consult them on the sort of clothes that will suit a particular occasion, whether I need a haircut, the box of chocolates which looks right for a present I want to give....
>
> A blind person should feel as much in a position as anyone else to

express his opinions and assert himself. But I often find it hard to take the initiative where another man would. If I am out with a girl shopping or hiking, when mealtime comes, I feel I must leave the choice of a cafe largely to her. Instead of saying, "I'm hungry! Let's go into the first cafe we find open," I will say, "Let's eat. But I'm afraid I will have to leave it to you to decide whether the first cafe we come to looks good enough." (Edwards, 1962, p. 86)

The end result of a reduced sense of competence is reduced self-esteem. The degree to which the blind person can (1) gather the requisite information himself, (2) make the necessary decisions himself, and (3) satisfactorily accomplish the tasks and activities without assistance is the degree to which he gains a sense of competence, of being in control of himself within his physical and social environment. "Improvements in the behavior of the visually impaired person will probably have a positive impact on the self-concept of the person independent of the attitudes and behaviors of others" (Welsh, 1980, p. 247).

Observed Performance

Significant others frequently are guilty of observing the behavior of blind persons more closely than they would that of others. As a result, many may be too quick to offer assistance, too cautious about perceived dangers, too fearful to permit mistakes or failures, and too impatient to allow the time required. In their eagerness to see VI succeed, they deprive him of the very building blocks required for later success.

Sometimes, there is a great deal of confusion about VI's performance of a given task. The extreme variability among visually impaired persons (see Chapter 1) produces apparently discrepant observations of performance. These inconsistencies may result from variations in degree of residual vision, fluctuations in vision, lighting conditions, distance, noise level, and/or familiarity with setting. Others observing VI frequently draw false conclusions from their apparent inconsistencies: "he's faking, he isn't really blind," "he's just lazy," "he's undependable."

The inner conflict and pathos are apparent in what on the surface seems to be a very humorous incident.

> To go back to my daylight experiences with the naked eye, it was me, in case you have heard the story, who once killed fifteen white chickens with small stones. The poor beggars never had a chance. This happened many years ago when I was living at Jay, New York. I had a vegetable garden some seventy feet behind the house, and the lady of the house had asked me to keep an eye on it in my spare moments and to chase away any chickens from neighboring farms that came pecking around. One morning, getting up from my typewriter, I wandered out behind the house and saw that a flock of white chickens had invaded the garden. I had, to be sure, misplaced my glasses for the moment, but I could still see well enough to let the chickens have it with ammunition from a pile of stones that I kept handy for the purpose. Before I could be stopped, I had riddled all the tomato plants in the garden, over the tops of which the lady of the house had, the twilight before, placed newspapers and paper bags to ward off the effects of frost. It was one of the darker experiences of my dimmer hours. (Thurber, 1937, p. 244)

Although not specifically expressed, feelings of embarrassment frequently result from inappropriate behaviors over which the visually impaired person has little or no control.

> Where we turned, I saw a moving form behind a wire fence and automatically raised my arm in neighborly greeting. It turned its profile to me and I saw a large, friendly horse. (Potok, 1980, p. 18)

Not all the significant others who happen to be noticing VI's performance will necessarily agree with each other about what they have observed. People tend to see what they want or expect to see. Similarly the observations of the significant others may not agree with VI's observations of his own behavior. VI may think he has accomplished a task, a conclusion not shared by others watching.

SELF-EVALUATION AND EVALUATION BY OTHERS

After the visually impaired person has engaged in the performance of an activity, VI and the observers make independent evaluations, either consciously or unconsciously,

regarding the extent to which the performance was satisfactory. People employ both community standards and
personal standards as yardsticks against which to measure
performance (James, 1890). The extent of the commonality
between community and personal standard will vary from
one individual to the next. For example, an individual's
standard of acceptable dress and appearance may or may
not agree with the commonly accepted community standards. The table etiquette in the Hocken family, where all
the members are visually impaired, may for practical
reasons differ from community standards.

> My consciousness of home centered on things like the smell of pies
> baking and the crackling sound of warmth of the fire, rather than its
> glow. When my family sat around the table for a meal and father asked
> someone to pass the salt, whoever traced his or her fingers across the
> tablecloth in search of it often knocked over a glass or bottle. But no
> one ever remarked about it. It was normal. My brother and I had no
> inkling that such mishaps did not occur in other households. (Hocken,
> 1977, p. 3)

Just as personal standards vary from one individual to
the next, so too community standards vary from one
referent group (comparison group) to the next. The community standard is the average of all the individual standards within that community. Part of the process of employing community standards is defining the community of
interest or identifying the relevant referent group. When the
community of interest is the wrestling team, then the
standard of acceptable strength may be quite different from
the standard of acceptable strength for another referent
group, such as band or French club.

When comparing the performance of an individual with
the community standard of some relevant referent group,
one can compare the performance with a perceived generalized standard or make social comparisons with specific
individuals within the relevant referent group. The choice of
the individual chosen as the basis for social comparison
becomes critical. If VI chooses to compare himself to the top
wrestler or the first chair trumpeter, then the evaluation
may be unfavorable. On the other hand, the results could

be quite different if the standard of social comparison were the last seated wrestler or the last seated trumpeter.

The standards of limits, according to Mangold (1982), enable an individual to evaluate his own performance and to determine growth in behavior and attitudes.

> They delineate areas of safety and danger, specify acceptable avenues through which to obtain goals, and enumerate the criteria that others use to judge success and failure. The handicapped child needs to learn that there is indeed a social reality that makes demands, provides rewards for accomplishments, and rejects those who do not demonstrate acceptable behavior. (p. 97)

Self-Evaluation

> This event [having some poems published] made no noticeable impact on the world of literature but it was quite the best thing which could have happened for me at that particular time. I began to feel that there were still some heights left to scale and many things worth doing. (Blackhall, 1962, p. 125)

Self-evaluation is the process of determining whether one's own performance is satisfactory or acceptable. For identical behaviors, judgments about acceptability will vary from one visually impaired person to another. Younger, less mature, and more dependent blind persons have a tendency to rely on social comparisons and community standards for their judgments about performance. More mature persons may develop internalized standards that are less susceptible to social comparisons and community standards.

The following illustration demonstrates the variability of acceptable standards. Most people take ten minutes to walk from a given location to the post office and back. One blind child making the trip in fifteen minutes may feel his performance is unsatisfactory because his teachers expect him to do it in ten. Another blind child making the trip in the same fifteen minutes may judge his performance to be acceptable because his best friend does it in twenty. A recently blinded adult may feel discouraged after making the trip in fifteen minutes because he is still employing community standards, whereas another individual, after a fifteen minute trip, may be pleased because he took five minutes off his previous time. Similarly, another individual may be pleased because he did something his significant others didn't expect him to accomplish.

> The formation of the self-concept depends upon two factors: 1. how a person perceives he is judged by significant others, and 2. a comparison of these judgments against a standard that he holds on how he should behave. Thus, his own judgment is constantly modified by his perception of the judgment of others. In other words, he is testing his perception against the reality of an external criterion. (LaBenne and Greene, 1969, p. 43)

It could be argued that, by lowering one's standards, more advantageous judgments of satisfactory or acceptable behavior would result in higher self-esteem. To continue the illustration used above, a person who is satisfied to complete a fifteen minute walk in twenty minutes has lowered his standard of acceptability, but since the task was accomplished successfully, his self-esteem should be increased. Coopersmith's (1967) study of preadolescent boys did not support this argument. "Persons with high self-esteem generally conclude they are closer to their aspirations than are the individuals with low self-esteem who have set lower goals" (p. 246). Higher self-esteem appears to be associated with striving for higher and higher standards of performance while being careful to keep the standard within reach.

Self-alienation begins to occur when one's behavior is unrelated to, or inconsistent with, his self-concept and personal aspirations.

> It seems more profitable, then, to view self-alienation as a noxious feeling arising when overt actions are detached or inconsistent with underlying conceptions of self. That is, self-alienation can be viewed as estrangement of the concept world from the daily activities of the individual. The individual might feel, "What I'm doing doesn't reveal the real me," "My behavior is a sham," or in its extreme form, "I hate what I do." (Gergan, 1971, p. 87)

Increased frustration and lowered self-esteem resulting from self-alienation processes are frequently experienced by newly blinded adults who are suddenly required to concentrate on relearning elemental skills which, until recently, were only incidentally related to his goals and aspirations.

My experiences are not unique. I had to learn to walk, to learn to feel for a desired object, to learn to recognize people by the sound of their voices. The casting out of former habits is perhaps more difficult than the acquiring of new ones. (Bretz, 1940, p. 185)

Evaluation by Others

At the same time that the visually impaired person is evaluating his own performance, the significant others, who have observed VI's behavior, are evaluating the acceptability of the performance. SO will, of course, use his own personal or referent group standards, rather than VI's set of standards. The extent to which SO's set of standards become imposed on VI or tend to dominate both evaluation processes is a function of the dependency of VI on SO.

During one's formative years, parents' standards dominate. Coopersmith (1967) suggested that explicit and enforced standards of conduct provide an adequate basis for judgments about the acceptability of one's behavior and, if unacceptable, exactly what corrections are necessary. He found that while explicit and enforced parental standards in preadolescent boys are associated with higher self-esteem children, uncertainty about standards seems to be related to the children's uncertain feelings of worth. This is particularly critical for those parents and teachers of visually impaired children who do not apply the same standard to VI as they do for others.

Unfortunately, when it comes to applying community standards to blind persons, all too often the community standards are abandoned in favor of specialized standards of behavior for "the blind." The tendency toward unique standards for the blind springs from latent or overt negative devaluating attitudes, as discussed in Chapter 3. The visually impaired person who senses that unique standards are being applied will feel cheated and devalued. This may result in a loss of self-esteem despite the good intentions of the significant other.

> A friend who lived next door dropped in one morning to say hello
> and found me busily engaged in making my bed for the first time. I
> refused the help offered, telling her I wanted to learn to do it myself,
> and we chatted while I finished. I asked her how it looked and she
> claimed it looked fine. After she left, Arnette [my sister] came in and
> said, "You've got the bedspread on upside down."
> "Why didn't she tell me?" I said furiously.
> "She said she didn't want to hurt your feelings."
> "But that's not helping me!" I retorted. (Carver, 1961, p. 163)

There are many opportunities for discrepancies to occur
among the evaluations of VI's performance, as seen in
Figure 11. VI's judgments may not concur with those of his
significant others. Furthermore, not all significant others
will agree with each other.

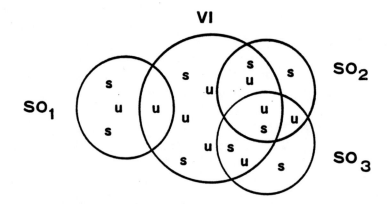

Figure 11. Judgments of Satisfactory (s) or Unsatisfactory (u) Performance

The availability of different sets of standards is another
potential source of discrepancy: personalized internal standards, community referent group standards, or unique
blindness standards. Similarly, the toleration of variability
in what one considers acceptable behavior varies a great
deal from one person to another. Certainly, the more the
evaluations of VI's performance differ from one another,
the less certain VI will be about his feelings of competence
and worthiness.

RESPONSES TO EVALUATIONS:
SUCCESS OR FAILURE

Evaluations of performance lead to judgments of success or failure. Attaining or exceeding aspirations or expectations is interpreted as success; falling short is interpreted as failure. "Our successes generally bring us recognition and are thereby related to our status in the community. They form the basis in reality for self-esteem and are measured by the material manifestations of success and by indications of social approval" (Coopersmith, 1967, p. 37).

James (1890) has interrelated self-esteem, success, and pretensions (a word he used for aspirations) in a formula: self-esteem = success/pretensions. "Such a fraction may be increased as well by diminishing the denominator as by increasing the numerator" (p. 310). In other words, self-esteem can be increased by either increasing the number of success experiences or by lowering aspirations or expectations . Fewer successes or lowered aspirations and expectations contribute to lowered self-esteem. "A child with low self-esteem is actually afraid of the obligation of living up to praise and of being successful. The person who believes in himself acts accordingly and puts forth effort to further his ends; but the person who depreciates himself sometimes gives up the struggle, and his performance as a consequence suffers" (Symonds, 1951, p. 88).

VI's Responses

The self-esteem of the person who is visually impaired is susceptible to judgments of success or failure. His own judgments of success in reaching his goals or the perceived judgments of success in reaching the expectations of others can reinforce his personal attributes, clarify his self-concept and improve his self-esteem. They provide the impetus to pursue even further aspirations and expectations in the same area. Krents discovered this when as a nine year old he played the violin for a Christmas concert.

[The lights dimmed] leaving the gym in complete darkness except for the hundred glimmering candles which were held by the choir as they softly sang the words of the carol from the balcony.

Slowly, and just as dramatically, the orchestra began to collapse in direct proportion to the dimming of the lights. When the lights went out completely, so did the orchestra, because no one could read his music—no one except me. My music stand had been totally unencumbered by music during the entire performance.

From the farthest corner of the stage, the sounds of one solitary but very proud second violinist filled the gymnasium. The choir and I went through verse after verse of the song, my confidence and happiness growing with each note. When it was all over, the ovation was positively thunderous. I sat back in my corner and let the waves of applause wash over me. Yes, even blindness has its compensations. (Krents, 1972, p. 122)

Sensitivity to failure varies a great deal from individual to individual. McAndrew (1948) studied self-predictions of hand strength using a hand dynamometer and found the blind children tested tended to be more sensitive than the sighted children to their failure to reach their previously estimated levels of aspirations. LaBenne and Greene (1969) suggested that some individuals "can accept failure without fear, while others fear to fail.... One defeat can appropriately be interpreted as 'I have failed' not 'I am a failure'" (pp. 12-13). Any person, whether blind or sighted, will be able to accept appropriate criticism without loss of self-esteem if he can offset his feelings of failure with the knowledge that there are many other things he can do well (Mangold, 1982). Occasionally, fear of failure is ungrounded.

This was my first attempt at a comeback since I had become blind, and the very thought of failure made me shiver.

An then I suddenly realized how foolish I was. These young people were probably just like the ones I had always known. . . . They could be depended upon to meet me halfway. I had been building up a wall between us, when all that I really had to do was to be honest with them. . . .

There was nothing prying about these questions. They were asked in an honest and respectful manner. . . . Nor was there the slightest note of pity. Here was someone who had solved a problem in which they were interested and they wanted to know how it was done. (Dahl, 1962, pp. 2, 6)

VI's possible responses to failure are numerous and may include one of the following:

1. Try harder: This response may take one of two forms. The individual can try harder by redoubling his efforts or he can try harder by finding a new way to circumvent the difficulty in order to accomplish the desired goal (Wright, 1960).

2. Alter aspirations: The individual can lower his aspirations to bring them more in line with his capacities. "With success his aspirations usually rise: with failure, they decline" (Wright, 1960, p. 92). On the other hand the individual may choose to substitute an attainable goal for the unattainable one and thereby achieve personal satisfaction.

3. Lower standards: Instead of striving to be the best, an individual can learn to be content with being "average," or he can compare his performance today with his own performance of yesterday, instead of employing a social comparison standard.

4. Give up: With repeated failures, one's efforts tend to diminish, assuring continued failure until, at last, all effort ceases. After a while, one begins to reason "with no attempt, there can be no failure; with no failure, no humiliation" (James, 1890, p. 310).

Just as repeated successes build expectations and patterns of future success, so do failures. When given the opportunity to demonstrate his ability, to assert himself, to offer leadership, the visually impaired person develops the confidence necessary for future successes. On the other hand, "not to believe that you are capable of success may actually guarantee your failure" (Gergan, 1971, p. 80).

SO's Responses

After the SO evaluates VI's performance, there is a judgment of the extent of success or failure in the attainment of SO's expectations. These judgments of success or failure affect the subsequent relationship between SO and

VI. Sometimes SO identifies so strongly with VI that SO's self-esteem fluctuates with VI's self-esteem. In any case, perceived success at meeting expectations reinforces SO's defining attributes of VI and subsequent expectations. SO's possible responses to perceived failure include providing remedial assistance, administering discipline, altering expectations, lowering standards, or giving up on VI.

During the process of formulating VI's and SO's responses to the judgments of success or failure, there are sources of potential discrepancies and misunderstandings. If VI judges his performance to be acceptable and he perceives SO altering aspirations, lowering standards, or even giving up on him, the blind person will be confused and may begin questioning his own judgments. Similarly if VI judges his performance to be unsatisfactory but SO judges it satisfactory, the significant other will not understand why VI persists pursuing a goal already attained.

A healthy self-esteem increases the likelihood of success, and success increases self-esteem. The converse is equally true for low self-esteem and failure. This principle is illustrated by Welsh (1980) in the area of mobility training for the blind.

> A positive self-concept can be both a cause and an effect of success in mobility.... If the person has developed a negative self-concept as a result of some of the natural reactions associated with visual loss in our culture, this attitude may reduce the likelihood that the person will aspire to achievement of success in independent travel. Either his poor self-concept prevents him from beginning the training, or his self-esteem will not sustain him through the initial frustrations and the anticipated fears. This lack of success will further reinforce his negative self-concept or result in some other defense mechanism that protects him from a negative self-evaluation.
>
> On the contrary, if the individual can be helped to experience success in the tasks of independent movement and can be rewarded for this success in the context of an accepting relationship with the mobility specialist, then perhaps the visually impaired person can begin to feel more positive about himself and continue to improve in these feelings throughout the training sequence. (pp. 226, 246)

Nonetheless, blind persons have just as much right to make mistakes and to fail as anyone else. They should not be shielded or protected from failing experiences. LaBenne and Greene (1969) felt that an individual can and ought to learn from his mistakes. Unfortunately, too often students get the impression that they should not make mistakes at school. On the contrary, students should be encouraged to explore many areas to discover their strengths and weaknesses, their interests and attitudes. At the same time "success has no substitute. Each person has a need to be successful. One cannot go through life being a failure at everything" (LaBenne and Greene, 1969, pp. 125-126).

Because of the cause and effect relationship between success and self-esteem, the pattern for this upward spiral should begin as early as possible. The confidence and self-esteem of a visually impaired child can be strengthened if during his school years he "has had enough time to complete his tasks and secure his objectives, so that by the time he reaches adolescence, he has behind him repeated experiences of achievement; a childhood history littered with unfinished tasks and unachieved goals can undermine this" (Chapman, 1978, p. 117).

VALUE PRIORITIES

"Each person has certain primary motivations or dominant values around which his self-system is organized. It is through the process of being internally consistent to those motivations and values that we can see overt expressions of behavioral consistencies" (Hamachek, 1971, p. 67). The significance of success or failure to the individual's self-esteem is not determined until the priority of the value it represents is known. If the success represents a high priority value in that individual's life, then the impact on his self-esteem is great. If the failure represents a low priority value, then the potential impact on self-esteem is negligible (James, 1890; Coopersmith, 1967).

Aspirations or expectations define the domain of VI's

performance. Certain standards are applied to that performance in order to make judgments about success or failure in reaching those aspirations or expectations. However, judgments of successful, acceptable behavior in and of themselves do not necessarily influence self-esteem in a positive direction. Only when the judgment of success is weighted by the relative priority of the value area the success represents will the extent of the positive influence on self-esteem be understood. "It is by living up to aspirations in areas that he regards as personally significant that the individual achieves high self-esteem" (Coopersmith, 1967, p. 37). Successfully conforming to expected social etiquette at the dinner table may have no impact on the self-esteem of a preadolescent boy for whom table manners happen to hold a very low priority. Nevertheless, it may have succeeded in improving the parent's self-esteem.

Of course, there is no uniform ranking of value priorities that would be acceptable to everyone. In addition, one's ranking of high priority values is not static, but is subject to change. However, there would undoubtedly be some tentative agreement about the relative importance of the following values: wealth, intelligence, spiritual growth, status, respect, happiness, health, pleasure, and appearance. Coopersmith (1967) defined areas of potential value to preadolescent boys as "the ability to influence and control others—which we shall term *Power*; the acceptance, attention, and affection of others— *Significance*; adherence to moral and ethical standards—*Virtue*; and successful performance in meeting demands for achievement—*Competence*" (pp. 38-39). He maintained that notable achievement in one of these four areas would result in higher self-esteem only if that area was regarded as important.

The following list includes some of the common high priority values frequently espoused by members of society. When these values are applied to VI, they may either consciously or unconsciously influence VI's self-esteem negatively.

1. "Olympic Gold Medalist": Body Whole
2. "Miss Universe": Body Beautiful

3. "But Everyone Else Does": Preoccupation with Normalcy or Conformity

4. "Just One of the Boys": Self-conscious Desire for Anonymity

5. "By the Sweat of My Brow": Work Ethic

6. "What Honors Have You Received": Competition for Achievement and Status

7. "I'd Rather Do It Myself": Self-sufficiency

8. "Please Don't Touch": Visually Oriented Society with Touch Taboos

9. "Where Did You Go On Vacation?": Mobile Society

10. "Have You Read the Current Best Seller?": Keeping Current and Up to Date

11. "One A Day Vitamin Supplements": Preoccupation with Health.

None of these values is necessarily undesirable in and of itself. However, when any of these values represents an exclusive or extreme priority for an individual, in an area void of recognition or success, it is likely to produce a lowering of self-esteem.

VI's Values

The values that are important in VI's life help him make decisions about choices among the many potential goals and activities. Some of the choices will represent valued areas that coincide with his capacities, thus increasing the likelihood of improving self-esteem. Pursuits in valued areas that, from the outset, have high probability of failure increase the likelihood of a negative impact on self-esteem.

"To know that someone considers himself inferior with respect to some particular quality is insufficient information to tell us what he thinks of himself. We must also have some idea of how much he *values* this quality" (Hamachek, 1971, p. 240).

If VI places a high priority on "body whole" and feels that it is best exemplified by members of the school football team, he may unconsciously devaluate himself for not being a member of the squad. For the individual who values "conformity." or "normalcy," the use of braille, long cane, and other special devices will result in lowered self-esteem. The person who values the ability to stay abreast of current events and literature will find it embarrassing and deflating to admit his deficiencies. When VI holds high priority values that place him at a disadvantage because of blindness, it tends to keep the disability at the focal point of attention.

SO's Values

The significant others will have their own independent set of values. Consequently, the weight or significance attached to VI's successes or failures will also be independently determined. SO who values body beautiful will consciously or unconsciously devaluate the person who happens to have disfigured eyes. Similarly, the significant other who places high priority on "self-sufficiency" will devaluate any manifestations of VI's dependence. In one way or another these high priority values are communicated to the blind person with their implied devaluating connotations, through SO's behavior, jokes, topics of conversation, stories about self, and anecdotes about others. Parents, teachers, and rehabilitation counselors must be careful about the unintended yet damaging message implied by their own value system.

Potential clashes between VI's values and SO's values provide another source for possible discrepancies. VI may not hold the same set of high priority values as his significant others, and the significant others' sets of values may not have much in common. It follows, therefore, that a particular success could be weighted heavily by one person and almost overlooked by another. Being able to use a closed circuit television reader may be viewed as a significant achievement by one person and as simply weird behavior by another. Conclusions about the impact on VI's self-esteem will vary depending on the significance attached by each person to each of VI's perceived successes and failures.

I subsequently procured a pair of glasses from their low visual aids department. They were weird-looking, and they made me look weird when using them. But I was far enough into the rehabilitation struggle that vanity was diminishing, and I did not much care what I looked like as long as I could try hard to overcome. (Kemper, 1977, p. 84)

BASIC DRIVES AND DEVELOPMENTAL NEEDS

Perhaps basic drives and developmental needs should have been discussed at the beginning of the chapter rather than at the end, as it is one's drives and needs that help to determine personal and defining attributes, aspirations and expectations, standards of evaluation, responses to success and failure, and priority values. However, the primary focus of this chapter is on development of self-esteem, not on development of the self. Premature discussion of drives and needs would have diverted attention away from the primary purpose.

Basic human drives motivate an individual to meet his perceived needs. The self is the mediator between one's drives and one's physical and social environment. Numerous words and phrases have been used by many different authors to describe these drives: self-preservation, self-seeking, self-appreciation (James, 1890); survival instinct (Cooley, 1902); superiority striving (Adler, 1927); self-realization, self-enhancement (Mead, 1934); self-affirmation, self-love (Fromm, 1939); self-sufficiency, security from anxiety, to be valued by self and others (Horney, 1945); to actualize, maintain, and enhance the self, self-acceptance (Rogers, 1951); self-actualization, reaching one's highest potential (Maslow, 1954); becoming fully functioning (Rogers 1961).

"Behavior is basically the goal-directed attempt of the organism to satisfy its needs as experienced, in the field as perceived" (Rogers, 1951, p. 491). These needs, which change as the organism grows and matures, are developmental in nature. The simplest developmental model describes the individual maturing from dependence to independence into interdependence. From the dependency of infancy, one grows into the independence of youth and adolescence, a period during which exploration, experimentation by trial and error, and testing limits prevail. The more mature recognize that interdependence is more satisfying to both self and others. There is a recognition that one cannot do everything for himself just as he cannot do nothing for himself (Rapp, 1974).

A more complex model of developmental needs was formulated by Erikson (1950). He described these needs as eight components of a healthy personality, which aggregate one upon the other. They are briefly described to show how one's personal attributes, aspirations, standards, and values are all influenced by one's particular level of development. The developmental stages are hierarchical. The ability of the child to develop trust is dependent upon the parent's level of ego integrity. The extent to which each succeeding need can be met is dependent upon the extent to which the preceding level was satisfied.

1. Trust: first 15 months.
   Characterized by maternal care, consistency, and continuity.
   Its opposite: basic mistrust.
2. Autonomy: 2-4 years of age.
   Characterized by a desire to do things himself; reassuring, firm outer control.
   Its opposite: shame and doubt.
3. Initiative: 5-6 years of age.
   Characterized by self-directed exploration, mutual regulation (child and parent).
   Its opposite: guilt.
4. Industry: 7-11 years of age.
   Characterized by recognition gained by producing things through use of skills and tools; models adult behavior.
   Its opposite: inferiority and inadequacy.
5. Identity: puberty and early adolescence.
   Characterized by questioning of sameness and continuities relied on earlier, sensitivity to peer pressure.
   Its opposite: role diffusion.
6. Intimacy: young adulthood.

Characterized by identification of self with people and things, ability to risk ego loss.
Its opposite: isolation.
7. Generativity: adulthood.
Characterized by ability to assume responsibility for own actions and for guiding next generation.
Its opposite: stagnation.
8. Ego integrity: maturity.
Characterized by the enjoyment of the fruit of the first seven stages; acceptance of one's one and only life cycle; organization of efforts toward integration.
Its opposite: despair, fear of death.

Although Erikson was referring to developmental levels he identified in the general population, they are also applicable to the segment of that population who happen to be blind. The visually impaired person's personal attributes, aspirations, standards, and values are all affected by his developmental level. The aspirations that VI establishes during "autonomy" differ from those established during "intimacy." The values employed during "trust" may differ from those employed during "industry."

Another model of developmental needs was developed by Maslow (1970). The model is hierarchical, that is, lower needs must be met before higher needs become salient. Again, it should be evident that an interaction is taking place between the developmental levels and one's personal attributes, aspirations, standards, and values.
1. Physiological needs: hunger and thirst.
2. Safety needs: security, protection, freedom from fear, anxiety and chaos.
3. Belongingness and love needs: affectionate and caring relations with people.
4. Esteem needs: desire for achievement, adequacy, and competence; desire for reputation, status, importance.
5. Need for self-actualization: doing what he individually is fitted for; fulfillment of one's highest potential.

As is true for all people, the blind person's level of development tends to define the domain of relevant personal attributes, aspirations, standards, and values. VI who is struggling with safety needs is unable to consider aspirations, standards, and values that are associated with esteem or self-actualization needs.

SUMMARY

The competence model of self-esteem presented in this chapter is more internally oriented than the social reflections model of the last chapter. However, reflections continue to play an important role in the competence model since they generate the data that stimulates further refinement of the self-concept and they provide additional sources of discrepancies between VI and SO. As was true of the process described in Chapter 4, the dynamic processes discussed in Chapter 5 are not unique to blindness, only intensified by blindness.

Two simultaneous cyclical sequences were developed in this chapter, both of which influence VI's self-esteem. From VI's point of view, the sequence moved from his personal attributes to the significance of his successes and failures, weighting the impact on self-esteem. From SO's frame of reference, the concurrent sequence moved from defining attributes to the priority values that weight his judgments of VI's successes and failures. The revised personal attributes encompass the new levels of VI's self-esteem, and the SO's defining attributes of VI encompass altered judgments of VI's value and worth. Because the sequence is cyclical, it would be helpful to represent the process in a circular diagram.

On each succeeding cycle either VI or SO or both may choose to alter any element of their respective processes. There are potential discrepancies (□) between VI and SO at every stage. (The resolution of these discrepancies is the topic of the next chapter.) When the processes converge in valued areas to produce failures as judged by VI or SO, then one's self-esteem is lowered. Successes and failures judged insignificant have little impact. Experiences that contribute to or result in successes in valued areas improve self-esteem.

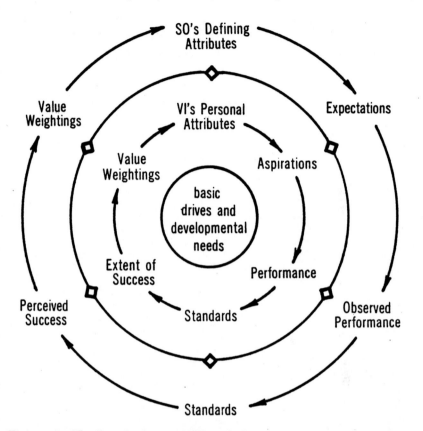

Figure 12. The Development of VI's Self-Esteem, a Sequential, Cyclical Model, Showing Interaction between VI and SO

It is natural and perhaps necessary for youth and some adults to seek the approval of others (Chapter 4) and to strive to prove their competence and worth to themselves and to others (Chapter 5). However, self-esteem that is built solely on reflected appraisals and competence is fragile, for people's feelings and attitudes are inconsistent and changeable and one's competence fluctuates with time, with the situation, and with the referent group. Sooner or later, an individual's self-esteem must be rooted in the fundamental position that he has dignity and worth simply because he is a person. When a person recognizes that he is of value not because of what he does or what other people say, but simply because he is a part of God's creation, a part of mankind, (Dobson, 1981), then he can quit the struggle to prove and to please, thus reducing the pressure, enabling him to be more fully self-actualized.

Chapter 6

SELF-ESTEEM AND THE
RESOLUTION OF DISCREPANCIES

L ife is a never-ending series of adjustments to new and different conditions for all people, whether blind or sighted. The child graduated from elementary school and entered junior high. Bobby just wrecked the family car. Mother had another baby. Father lost his job. Grandfather died. The new and different conditions affect not only the individual but also his significant others.

Consistency, unity, and stability are among the properties of the self and self-concept presented in Chapter 4. A person usually behaves in a manner consistent with his self-concept. The global self strives for consistency and unity. The self-concept, although subject to modification, is resistant to change. "Because the self-concept shapes new experience to conform to its already established pattern, much behavior can be understood as a person's attempt to maintain the consistency of his self concept, a kind of homeostasis at a higher psychological level" (Shaffer and Shoben, 1956, p. 94).

Each new and different condition becomes another threat to this psychological homeostasis. The interaction of the person who is visually impaired (VI) with his social and physical environment provides many opportunities for clashes, discrepancies, and dissonance (see Chapter 5). Cognitive dissonance is the mingling of discrepant ideas and behaviors and results in discomfort, conflict, and tension (Hamachek, 1971). "The presence of dissonance gives rise to pressures to reduce or eliminate the dissonance. The strength of the pressures to reduce the dissonance is a function of the magnitude of the dissonance" (Festinger, 1962, p. 18).

To the extent that discrepancies threaten to expose an individual's inadequacies, they are anxiety-arousing. Physiological tension, psychological discomfort, and anxiety result when an individual perceives himself as unacceptable to himself, unworthy of respect, having to live by the standards of others (Rogers, 1961). Anxiety and self-esteem are closely yet inversely related: the higher the anxiety, the greater the threat to self-esteem.

The self-preserving and self-protective drives motivate a person to mobilize his resources to deal with the threats. "The self-system is an organization of educative experience called into being by the necessity to avoid or to minimize incidents of anxiety" (Sullivan, 1953, p. 165). There is a natural healthy tendency for a person to maintain stablity and harmony, to minimize anxiety and conflict, to reduce discrepant and dissonant ideas and behaviors.

> A person cannot remain in an extreme state of disequilibrium, and a crisis is thus, by definition self-limited. Within a few days or weeks some resolution, even though temporary, must be found, and some equilibrium reestablished. The new balance achieved may represent a healthy adaptation which promotes personal growth and maturation, or a maladaptive response which signifies psychological deterioration and decline. (Moos and Tsu, 1977, p. 7).

However, not all conflicts or tensions are necessarily bad. If VI relates only with persons whose defining attributes (DA), expectations, standards, and values agree with his own personal attributes (PA), aspirations, standards, and values, then he is seldom challenged to reevaluate his self-concept. Significant others' (SO) expectations of VI that are higher than his own aspirations undoubtedly cause anxiety and friction but, if not so extreme as to be debilitating, may also motivate to greater successes and higher self-esteem.

Similarly, VI's apparently discrepant behaviors are not always detrimental. They do not necessarily indicate that his inconsistent actions stem from a fragmented self-concept. Observing apparent discrepant behavior may simply mean that the observer has failed to recognize the deepest or most salient motives that are operating in the visually impaired person's life (Hamachek, 1971).

SOURCES OF DISCREPANCIES AND ANXIETIES

Anxiety is a common experience. Children are especially vulnerable to the whims of a potentially hostile world and frequently experience feelings of insecurity and inadequacy (Horney, 1945). Among the numerous factors contributing to anxiety in all children, as discussed by Horney, are isolation from other children, overprotection, lack of real guidance, domination, disparaging devaluating attitudes, indifference and lack of respect, too much or too little admiration, too much or too little responsibility, lack of reliable consistent warmth, and being discriminated against. It is appalling to observe how many of these factors were discussed in Chapters 2 and 3 as particular problems for blind children and adults alike.

As has already been noted, the self can manifest itself in many ways, each with its own uniqueness but not necessarily compatible with the other selves. The following are a few of the possible "selves":

1. the subjective self: what VI thinks himself to be, his personal attributes.
2. the presented self: the way VI presents himself.
3. the objective self: VI's factual behavioral, physical, and psychological characteristics and traits.
4. the ideal self: what VI wants to become.
5. the potential self: what VI could become within the limits of the projected capacities.
6. the moral self: what VI ought to be, morally and ethically.
7. the fantasized self: VI's "if only" magic wand, wishful dreams.
8. the perceived self: VI as defined by others, the defining attributes.

9. the expected self: VI as defined by others' expectations.
10. the compliant self: the extent to which VI meets others' expectations.

These selves may clash with each other at various times and in various settings, producing unnecessary conflicts and tensions. The following illustrates the clash between the ideal self and the objective self.

> Thurber's nastiness, I suppose, was because of his blindness. He wanted to see the same things as everybody else. He was not a good blind man, and he never really got used to it. He liked to believe he could see more than he actually could. When I drove for him, he would like to start the car. I would sit behind the wheel patiently while he pushed and twisted the cigarette lighter or the wiper switch, thinking they were the ignition. I guess I was no different from many other people in Cornwall who humored him only because he was blind and famous. (Bernstein, 1975, p. 379)

Whenever there is a reputation to be upheld, one can question whether the presented self is the same as the actual self.

> My wrestling and beer drinking had defined me as a certain kind of person—the Joe College sort. I had to preserve this reputation and, if possible enlarge upon it, or at least fill in the details. (Russell, 1962, pp. 108-109)

As with Kemper, many blind individuals find that their subjective self stands in sharp contrast to their perceived self.

> The partially sighted person encounters a different, more insidious, prejudice. In the case of a person who sees everything in general but nothing in particular, one's fellow human beings feel deceived. Others know of my visual loss, but when they hear that I play golf (no matter how ineptly) or that I function as senior minister of a large congregation, they are surprised and confused over their expectations of who I am and what I can or cannot do. (Kemper, 1977, p. 102)

Each of these selves may manifest themselves differently in one's various settings: home, school, office, church, club. Most self-concept measures focus on the discrepancy between the subjective self (one's perception of what he is) and the ideal self (what one wants ideally to be). "Most research evidence indicates that people who are highly self-critical

—that is, who show a large discrepancy between the way they actually see themselves and the way they would ideally like to be—are less well-adjusted than those who are at least moderately satisfied with themselves" (McCandless, 1967, p. 280).

The possibilities of other discrepancies are numerous, as discussed throughout Chapters 4 and 5. A summary of the potential discrepancies might include the following:

1. For the visually impaired person and a significant other—
   a. between VI's PA and SO's DA, subjective vs. perceived self;
   b. between VI's aspirations and SO's expectations, ideal vs. expected self;
   c. between VI's performance and his observed performance by SO;
   d. between VI's standards and SO's standards;
   e. between VI's responses and SO's responses to successes and failures;
   f. between VI's values and SO's values;
   g. between subjective self and expected self;
   h. between subjective self and compliant self.
2. For VI's significant others—
   a. among their DA's, their perceived selves;
   b. among their expectations, their expected selves;
   c. among their observed performances;
   d. among their standards;
   e. among their responses to VI's successes and failures;
   f. among their value priorities;
   g. among their compliant selves.
3. Within VI himself—
   a. between PA and aspirations, subjective vs. ideal self;
   b. between aspiration and performance, ideal vs. objective self;
   c. between performance and standards, measure of success;
   d. between performance and values, objective vs. moral self;

e. between objective self and subjective self;
f. between subjective self and potential self;
g. between ideal self and compliant self.

Really sharp differences between one's self-concept and what one wants to be (the ideal self) are related to personal unhappiness. There is also evidence that excessive self-satisfaction (no difference between the perceived and the ideal self) has its disadvantages. A certain amount of restless discontent or dissatisfaction may act as a constructive force (ambition) urging individuals to better themselves. (McCandless, 1977, p. 522)

The process of recognizing and accommodating to the many contradictions and inconsistencies in life's experiences is the same for both blind and sighted persons. Visually impaired children and adults encounter the same kind of discrepancies experienced by everyone else. However, blindness tends to exacerbate the discrepancies, especially in situations where blindness is perceived as such a significant factor that it becomes the focal point of understanding and interpreting all behavior.

REACTIONS TO DISCREPANCIES

It is no wonder that VI may have some difficulties sorting out all the contradictory messages from without and conflicting perceptions from within. Because the perceptions of the significant others are frequently discrepant among themselves, the extent of the discrepancy between VI and SO will vary from one significant other to the next. Frequent and persistent inconsistencies lead to a poor self-concept. "Any experience which is inconsistent with the organization or structure of self may be perceived as a threat, and the more of these perceptions there are, the more rigidly the self-structure is organized to maintain itself" (Rogers, 1951, p. 515).

The visually impaired person's limited access to nonverbal communication may produce even further uncertainties. Facial expressions, gestures, and body language provide important signals that may not be perceived by the visually impaired person. When VI perceives cues either from within or from the significant others that are ambiguous and vague, he will use his memory for supporting collaborative evidence. However, since memory is selective, there is a tendency for the individual to remember only those experiences that provide positive confirmation of his own biases (Gergan, 1971).

Persons with high self-esteem tend to respond to contradiction and inconsistencies more realistically than persons with low self-esteem (Coopersmith, 1967). With their histories of successes, they have developed a confidence in their own abilities and judgments, and this confidence produces a greater likelihood of further successes.

> On the other hand, we must also recognize that it really is possible for a person to be totally disabled by his negative self-concept. Under these circumstances, there is relatively little one can do, because no amount of assurance, no discussion of his abilities and worth can convince him that he has a chance for success. His logic allows him to find proof for his assumptions of failure, and objective reality is no match for what he *believes* himself to be. In other words, once a person has a conviction, he finds the experiences necessary to support this conviction. Furthermore, since perception is selective, he tends to perceive only those things which support his beliefs and ignores those which are contrary to his assumptions. (LaBenne and Greene, 1969, p. 123)

An individual can be perceived as a failure in one setting and as quite successful in another. He can be quite confident in one situation while feeling totally inadequate in another. In certain circumstances he may tend to be submissive, while in others he may tend to dominate or exert leadership. A person usually has multiple roles, multiple selves, multiple parts of the global self. The integration of new information about the self is not necessarily required at the global level. It is sufficient that it be integrated at the parts level (Wright, 1960).

"We may conclude then, that inconsistencies in the concepts of self may be perfectly natural and wide-spread. At the same time there may be a generalized tendency to reduce inconsistency" (Gergan, 1971, p. 22). The strength of this tendency is a function of (1) the awareness of the inconsistencies by the people involved, (2) the clash of opposing views in the same setting, (3) the functional value of the discrepancy to each, and (4) the learned capacity to avoid inconsistencies (Gergan, 1971).

THE RESOLUTION OF DISCREPANCIES

Rogers, Horney, Arkoff, and Wright each described their own views regarding the manner by which people resolve discrepancies.

Rogers (1951) described three possible responses to encounters with one's social and physical environment. "As experiences occur in the life of the individual, they are either (a) symbolized, perceived, and organized into some relationship to the self, (b) ignored because there is no perceived relationship to the self-structure, (c) denied symbolization or given a distorted symbolization because the experience is inconsistent with the structure of the self" (p. 503).

According to Horney (1945), people handle contradictions within themselves by (1) "moving toward people"— compliant, dependent, helpless; (2) "moving away from people"—detached, independent, isolated; or (3) "moving against people"—competitive, aggressive, hostile (p. 42).

Arkoff (1968) suggested five ways to cope with contradictions and inconsistencies: (1) restructure, giving each child his own bedroom reduces conflict; (2) compromise, both parties move toward an acceptable middle ground; (3) accommodation, the parties involved learn to tolerate the problem; (4) mediation, the parties involved seek professional help; and (5) escape, one or both individuals leave (pp. 335-339).

Yet another point of view is presented by Wright (1960). "It is disturbing to the subject when his expectations do not match the presenting facts, and he feels the need to reconcile the two. This may be accomplished by such cognitive changes as *expectation revision, altering apparent reality and anormalizing the person*" (p. 73).

Although the following discussion is applied specifically to the visually impaired, it should not be assumed that the process is unique to the blind. Elements of the four models just presented are incorporated into the following discussion. Perhaps, out of necessity, persons who are blind learn to tolerate greater and more frequent contradictions and inconsistencies than do the sighted. In general, when VI encounters discrepancies among his significant others, he will either accept the opinions that are closest to his own or he will revise his own opinions in favor of the most credible, the most respected and reliable, the most caring and accepting, the most persistent and frequent, or the most positive.

Resolving Discrepancies by Unilateral Revisions

The visually impaired person may, when confronted by a strong dominating significant other, repress or relinquish his own personal attributes, aspirations, standards, evaluations, and/or values and adopt SO's defining attributes, expectations, standards, evaluations, and/or values as his own. Children particularly are vulnerable to strong domination by others. Dependent adults as well seek their security by compliance.

> It came in a flash. Mr. Humphrey had been trying to impress upon me how a blind man could adjust himself to a guide dog. I had been thinking in terms of how a dog could be molded into a guide for a blind man, but I had not truly identified myself with that blind man. I had been trying to think as an instructor, making the whole thing into a sort of intellectual game, mathematical, rigid and absolute. I wanted rational explanations for everything. . . .
>
> My blindness, the very first thing upon which Mr. Humphrey had laid his emphasis, must be a perpetual unknown in the guide-dog equation, and having fully recognized this fact for the first time, I began to see. (Putnam, 1952, pp. 103-104)

At the same time, SO may, in the face of a strong self-assured blind person, repress or relinquish his own defining attributes, expectations, standards, evaluations, and/or values. In this situation, it is apparent that VI must be assertive and possess a fairly well-defined self-concept. It also presumes that SO is secure enough to be willing to alter his opinions about VI. On the other hand, it may mean that SO is compliant and dependent by nature. With a little convincing, Davey's grandparents were able to alter their defining attributes.

> They marveled at his ability to get around. In spite of all we had told them, they could not think of him walking alone. It had seemed to them, in their thoughts of him, that he would have to be led everywhere. His independence was like a sort of miracle to them. They followed him as he went about the house, watching with anxiety and delight his maneuvering of doorways and turns. That first day taught them many, many things. They had not known, until then, that Davey's blindness was only a part of him, not the whole. Before that, they had thought of him as a blind child. Now they thought of him as a lovable child who, incidentally, was blind. It was a very different way of thinking. (Henderson, 1954, pp. 117-118)

Unilateral revisions have an effect on VI's feelings about himself. Self-esteem will be improved when the adopted elements of the process are more positive and approving than the relinquished. On the other hand, if the adopted elements are more devaluating and disapproving than the relinquished, then VI's self-esteem will suffer.

Resolving Discrepancies by Mutual Revisions

Mutual revisions are probably the most common process of reducing contradictions and inconsistencies. It involves VI and SO both moving toward more mutually agreeable or tolerable positions regarding personal and defining attributes, aspirations and expectations, standards, evaluations and/or values. For VI, it means retaining a few ideas, giving up others, and compromising on still others. After the revisions, the relationship is more likely to be harmonious, providing a healthy climate for mutual growth in self-esteem. In the following excerpt, the dog guide, Hank, became the catalyst that brought VI and her acquaintances closer together.

> People's attitudes are funny things, sighted and blind. I've lived in my building for seven years. Before I got my dog, Hank, six years ago, I think five people in the building would say hello to me, out of four or

five hundred tenants. I would walk in the neighborhood and very few people would say hello, goodbye, go to hell. Partly it was my fault because I'm Miss Independence; partly it was because people were not quite sure about how to deal with me. But since I've had Hank, I get stopped by absolute strangers. I get Good Morning, Hello, How Are You, Where's the Dog, I haven't seen you for a couple of days. A kind of attitude that people never had before. (Sperber, 1976, p. 235)

Resolving Discrepancies by Suppressing the Facts

For the sake of what he considers a more comfortable relationship, VI may choose not to divulge all the facts. When the individual who is visually limited meets someone whose attitudes toward blindness are either unknown or known to be disparaging, VI is frequently tempted to withhold the information that he himself is blind. If there is in fact, pretence involved, that is, VI is pretending to be sighted, then he is said to be playing the game Wright (1960) called "as if." He is playing "as if" he were sighted. This game is indicative of low self-esteem, for the motivation to play the game is rooted in VI's own disparaging attitudes toward blindness. He is seeking to hide something of which he is ashamed.

I do remember holding books very close to my face. When my teachers would call on me to get up and read something they would always say, "Take that book from your face!"

As a child, I would not admit that I had a problem. I had a pair of glasses that were given to me at one time but they were of absolutely no benefit. I was terribly vain so I just didn't bother with them. My social life was not impaired by this condition. . . .

As a girl at that time I wanted to write a book called "Blind Girl's Bluff" because I had discovered there were thousands of ways to avoid letting people know that I had this terrible affliction. I was aware of what was wrong with me but I did not want to admit it. If I was meeting a new fellow, he wasn't going to know for anything. I pretended I had to hold his hand because of a mysterious feeling that I would get. He, of course, would not object. . . . I never went out on a date feeling relaxed as a normal girl would. (Sperber, 1976, p. 38)

Suppressing the facts is not always done at the conscious level. VI's behavior however may reveal that he is playing "as if."

Helen [Thurber's wife] remembered that she would often see her husband alone in his working room just scribbling away meaninglessly on pieces of yellow copy paper. "He needed to perform the physical act of writing," she said. (Bernstein, 1975, p. 386)

In contrast to "as if," there are situations when VI may choose to "pass," when disclosure or nondisclosure about one's blindness is irrelevant. Although Goffman (1963) described a broader range of behaviors as "passing," his description included "accidental" and "unintentional" passing. VI "passes" when telephoning an order to the catalogue department, because the fact that he is blind is not relevant. In fact, to identify himself as blind would indicate an unhealthy fixation on blindness. It should be obvious that one could never "pass" in a lasting relationship with a significant other.

[During a sight reading band contest] we took our seats, and when the judges were ready, Mr. Welch was allowed a few minutes to review with us a few things about the key signatures and rhythm changes in the piece of music we were about to play. Then we began, and in a short time, it was all over. All I remembered was putting the saxophone to my lips and pressing a few keys up and down. I was afraid to make any noise for fear that I might play a note that was so far off it would bring the judges to our section immediately. What would they say if they knew that George Washington High School's first chair tenor saxophone player never blew one note? They could have slapped a piece of blank typewriter paper in front of me on the music stand and I would have done just as well. (Cordellos, 1981, p. 12)

In the same way, the significant other may choose not to disclose certain information because of potential discrepancies with VI. SO might choose to withhold some particular discrepant defining attribute or expectation that, if disclosed, would create conflict and tension. Although this appears to be hypocritical, it may be done for the sake of harmony.

Resolving Discrepancies by Restructuring the Situation

Sometimes the easiest way to reduce conflict and tension is to restructure the situation to prevent or minimize the clashing of two discrepant points of view. For example, there are blind children who have been moved from unaccepting, devaluating classrooms because the teacher's negative attitude would not or could not be revised. An employer, who senses a conflict errupting, may move an unaccepting employee out of VI's department.

Resolving Discrepancies by Selective Scanning

Selective scanning is the process of actively seeking, picking, and choosing the stimuli that are supportive or confirmatory, while ignoring the discrepant. "The mechanism of selectivity is such that it operates to help shape our self-attitudes in accord with our desires and in line with our strengths" (Hamachek, 1971, p. 247). People tend to see what they want to see and hear what they want to hear. This process tends to maintain an individual's self-esteem at a fairly constant level, whether positive or negative, unless something drastic or unusual happens.

Selective scanning that is used to support unrealistic attributes, aspirations, or expectations results in a distorted self-concept. However, selective scanning is not always detrimental and in some instances may be essential for success. For example, VI may choose to ignore those who would discourage him, those who have misgivings about his abilities, those who believe he cannot succeed, and continue to pursue his own aspirations based on other feedback that is more positive.

Now that I am a practicing doctor, I still run into doubters. Among patients. Among my fellow professionals. On some bad days I'm one of them. Every doubter I run into brings me down a notch. But after the blues of slipping a few notches, something stirs up the recollection of all the past discouragers and doubters, the ones who said I shouldn't, or couldn't, study science in high school or college because I'd only fail; the ones who said that even if I could qualify I wouldn't be accepted by a medical school; the ones who warned me against the relentless competition of National Board exams that med students have to survive over and over again (and many don't).

At some point you just tire of doubters and doubting, and you want to just walk away from them and get on with it. (Hartman and Asbell, 1978, p. 10)

Resolving Discrepancies by Distorting the Facts

Perceptions are subject to interpretations and, of course, misinterpretations. One way to circumvent potential discrepancy is to give the contradictory perception another meaning that is more satisfying or harmonious. Some sighted individuals expect blind persons to behave in certain ways and when VI doesn't, the facts are distorted to avoid expectation discrepancy. Fitting the facts to one's expectations sometimes requires him to impute special gifts or abilities to explain unexpected behavior that, nevertheless, is really quite ordinary and routine. "Selective interpretation of the facts, then, is one way of maintaining and enhancing a positive self-image" (Hamachek, 1971, p. 242). In the following excerpt a passerby selectively interpreted and distorted the facts by concluding that Anne really had nothing wrong with her vision.

> Anne, aged seven, and I were walking down the street holding hands. As we were crossing a side street she slipped off the pavement, and although I warned her she tripped up the opposite curbstone. A passer-by showed concern and whispered, "Can't she see?" I shook my head and she looked suitably sorry. Then Anne, safely on the pavement, cocked her head on one side, stood still, and using the very limited sphere of vision in her one eye said in a loud, clear voice, "Is that a girl driving the milk van?" The woman looked furious and stumped away. I felt guilty and ashamed, but, short of involving the child in a long embarrassing discussion, how could I explain that sometimes, if she was in the right position, she saw something quite clearly, but she couldn't look down at her feet? (Lunt, 1965, pp. 33-34)

Sometimes distorting the facts takes the form of blaming blindness for all of VI's failures or mistakes, as Hartman did when a girl he had been dating began to show interest in another fellow.

> It was one of those moments—and they have recurred since—when I found myself strangely grateful that I was blind. My blindness had to be the reason she was treating me like an unfeeling thing, like dirt, like nothing. If it couldn't be blamed on that, it had to be blamed on me. And that would have been unbearable. (Hartman and Asbell, 1978, pp. 74-75)

Resolving Discrepancies by Escape

If the discrepancies and conflicts persist and there seems to be no other resolution possible, then either VI or SO may attempt to escape the conflict. This can be accomplished either by physically leaving the scene or by psychologically withdrawing. Under extreme pressures and unusual circumstances, escape may take the form of suicide. Escape may bring about a reduction in tension and conflict but the impact on self-esteem is negative because of perceived failure or rejection.

> In all my shopping expeditions I have known nothing but kindness except in one instance. This occurred in the shop of a tailor who was fitting a suit for me. When I firmly refused to give in on one detail, he burst out impatiently, "Oh, why should you care—you can't see it anyway." I reminded him that my husband and friends could see it and I like them to be pleased. I let him finish the work but, unwilling to risk a repetition of such an incident, I have never returned to his shop. (McCoy, 1963, p. 66)

While the above anecdote illustrates VI's escape, when she refused to return to the tailor shop, the following escape was accomplished by a significant other.

> In less than two years Mike went from being the professional golfer to enrolling at our training center. In that time span he lost his sight from diabetes, had to give up driving and received a divorce notice from his wife because she, in her words, "Could not be married to a vegetable." (Fries, 1980, p. 369)

Successful resolution of discrepancies between VI and SO is not always possible. In this case there are two alternatives. Some people simply learn to tolerate the discrepancies and learn to live with the resultant conflicts and tensions.

> The first rule, I decided was that I must be true to myself. I must do the best job possible, and not allow my handicap to stand in my way. I, more than anyone else, knew my true self. I must live up to that self, and not to what people expected of me. Because of my blindness, people expected less from me than I knew I could give (Brown, 1958, p. 184)

On the other hand, one or both of the parties when they feel threatened may begin to employ psychological defense mechanisms.

DEFENSE MECHANISMS

In each of the methods for resolving conflict, the stimuli producing the discrepancy can be either positive or negative and the results have a chance of being constructive. Defense mechanisms, however, are employed either consciously or unconsciously in response to negative or devaluating stimuli and, being defensive, do not permit growth, only retreat and retrenchment. Defensive reactions are learned behaviors and require a certain amount of self-deception. They are used to reduce anxiety and to preserve one's self-esteem.

> In the study of how the personality functions, this ability to maintain self-esteem in the face of negative appraisals and discomfiture has been described by such concepts as controls and defenses. These terms refer to the individual's capacity to define an event filled with negative implications and consequences in such a way that it does not detract from his sense of worthiness, ability, or power. (Coopersmith, 1967, p. 37)

Defensive mechanisms include a wide range of behaviors familiar to every psychologist. Some of the more common are denying disagreeable reality, identifying for vicarious satisfaction, compensating for weakness by emphasizing strength, somatizing one's anxieties into physical ailments, internalizing threatening situations, malingering to avoid the unwanted, lying to cover inadequacies or failures, regressing to a former safe state, displacing of strong emotion onto a more neutral person or object, repressing of painful or dangerous thoughts, rationalizing to excuse behavior, projecting blame onto others, and fantasizing a desirable dream world.

It is natural and normal for people to use a few defensive reactions occasionally; however, extensive use is an indicator of poor adjustment and low self-esteem. Prevention of low self-esteem along with its need to utilize defense mechanisms is accomplished by developing and maintaining good mental health. Stringer (1971) discussed four psycho-social resources that will enable an individual to respond to stress more effectively: good interpersonal relationships; a healthy self-esteem; competence, productivity, and responsibility; and a large capacity for enjoyment.

CHARACTERISTICS OF HIGH AND LOW SELF-ESTEEM

Everyone experiences intra- and inter-personal discrepancies and all share the need to resolve them. However, not all manage the dissonance in the same way nor with the same degree of effectiveness. Persons with positive self-appraisal, healthy self-concept, high self-esteem, and good mental health are able to respond to and cope with the inevitable discrepancies much more effectively than low self-esteem persons.

Adler (1927) has indicated that feelings of inferiority are a universal experience. "Most teenagers decide they are without human worth when they're between thirteen and fifteen years of age" (Dobson, 1978, p. 16). However, the degree and intensity of these feelings vary a great deal among children, teenagers, and adults.

Throughout Chapters 4, 5, and 6, there are references to high and low self-esteem along with a discussion of some of the factors that impact on self-esteem. With this background, it is appropriate to summarize from the literature many of the characteristics of high self-esteem persons and also characteristics of low self-esteem persons. Some of the authors (Jourard, 1959; Maslow, 1970; Rogers, 1961; Wright, 1960) focused more on adults, while others (Coopersmith, 1967; Dobson, 1975; Horney, 1945; Rosenberg, 1965) focused much more exclusively on children and youth. The following summary represents some of the characteristics that appear to be generalizable to the preadolescent, adolescent, and adult populations. A person with high self-esteem does not necessarily exhibit all or even most of the qualities listed. On the other hand, a person exhibiting a few of the following characteristics does not necessarily possess high self-esteem.

Characteristics of High Self-esteem

1. Persons with high self-esteem tend to identify with their parents because during their childhood they—
   a. had mothers who exhibited higher levels of self-esteem and emotional stability and manifested more realistic orientation toward life;
   b. had closer relationships with their fathers;
   c. experienced parental acceptance (i.e. parental respect, care, concern, and attention) and parental receptivity to individual expression and dissent, within clearly defined limits that were consistently and strictly enforced;
   d. gained confidence in their own abilities through positive parental expectations;
   e. recognized that strong decision-making authority rested consistently with either the mother or the father but was not shared by both simultaneously.
2. Persons with high self-esteem tend to possess the intrapersonal characteristics described as—
   a. respecting, trusting, and accepting self, with an appropriate appreciation and love of self;
   b. avoiding undue worry about tomorrow's problems, today's events, or yesterday's mistakes;
   c. being more self-directed, being guided by their own standards and values rather than continually striving to meet cultural expectations, standards, and values;
   d. guiding their behavior by a well-developed sense of ethics;
   e. having confidence in their own perceptions and judgments, enabling them to be more creative and spontaneous;
   f. expecting to be successful in their endeavors and expecting to be well received by others;
   g. exhibiting less self-conscious behavior and less preoccupation with personal problems;
   h. showing an unhostile sense of humor;
   i. being relatively content with their situation;

    j. having a continuing appreciation for the good things in life and enjoying themselves in a wide variety of activities;

    k. needing periods of privacy that provide time for intense concentration on personal interests;

    l. being able to adapt to change, open to new experiences, and continually engaged in a growth process.

3. Persons with high self-esteem tend to possess the interpersonal characteristics described as—

    a. being sensitive to the needs of others;

    b. considering themselves of interest and value to others;

    c. feeling equal to others as a person irrespective of abilities, background, or appraisals of others;

    d. being more independent, and being less susceptible to others' attempts to influence them;

    e. accepting criticism more readily, and accepting praise and compliments without false modesty and guilt;

    f. being more realistic in response to devaluating appraisals;

    g. in general, not retreating behind a facade, but being consistent in social behavior and, more specifically, tending to disclose themselves fully to at least one other person;

    h. accepting their physical and social environment, particularly appreciating others as individuals without prejudice;

    i. manifesting a broad concern for the welfare of mankind;

    j. judging themselves to be competent relative to members of their group, tending to experience greater numbers of successes in areas that are important to them;

    k. taking more active and assertive roles in social groups;

    l. having less difficulty in forming friendships and the relationships formed are deeper;

    m. receiving from significant others respect, acceptance, and concerned treatment, being treated as a person with dignity, value, and worth;

n. giving and productive yet able to receive in return.

Characteristics of Low Self-esteem

1. Persons with low self-esteem tend to recall less than satisfactory relations with their parents because during their childhood they—

   a. were more often rejected and frequently viewed as a failure, resulting in lack of confidence, submission, withdrawal, and diminished effort, or aggressive and domineering behavior;

   b. had mothers with low self-esteem who were dissatisfied;

   c. observed extensive conflict between mother and father;

   d. experienced extended absences of the father from the home;

   e. were confused by decision-making authority shared equally by mother and father;

   f. lacked definite rules and limits and experienced inconsistent and severe punishment.

2. Persons with low self-esteem tend to possess the intrapersonal characteristics described as—

   a. being more dependent, accommodating and compliant, striving to please others, and striving to conform passively to the prevailing demands of the physical and social environment;

   b. experiencing high anxiety, frustration, distress, and a sense of inadequacy because of demands they cannot meet, and more frequently encountering failure;

   c. possessing inferiority feelings, timidity, self-alienation, lack of self-acceptance;

   d. exhibiting a basic disparaging and hostile attitude toward life;

   e. setting lower aspirations and diminished expectations for success;

   f. lacking trust in themselves and in their own perceptions and judgments and thus reluctant to express unpopular opinions;

   g. being preoccupied with personal problems and difficulties;

   h. feeling they are not of value, feeling unloved, unlovable, lonely, and sad;

   i. finding their security by returning to earlier behavior patterns.

3. Persons with low self-esteem tend to possess the interpersonal characteristics described as—

   a. experiencing social isolation and poor peer relationships, greater difficulty and hesitation in social interactions;

   b. feeling self-conscious, preferring a passive, silent role in a group, and the protection of anonymity;

   c. demonstrating a reluctance to engage in competition;

   d. avoiding the disclosure of self to others, thus avoiding exposure of weaknesses and inadequacies;

   e. exhibiting a hypercritical attitude, thus redirecting attention away from their own weaknesses;

   f. excusing their own weaknesses by blaming others;

   g. being sensitive to criticism, over-reacting to flattery and praise;

   h. using inappropriate defense mechanisms when threatened by devaluating stimuli;

   i. possessing feelings of paranoia, and persecution complex;

   j. having a self-esteem that is much more dependent on the reflected appraisals of others;

   k. being insensitive to the needs of others.

Characteristics of high and low self-esteem are just as evident among visually impaired children and adults as they are in the rest of the population. Some of the characteristics described have implications for parents. The intrapersonal and interpersonal attributes provide some guidelines for the professional to develop activities that encourage high self-esteem and its resultant behaviors.

SUMMARY

The process of recognizing and dealing with contradictions and inconsistencies is the same for both blind and sighted. The self may manifest itself in many different ways at different times, in various situations. Although the global self strives for consistency and unity, a certain number of contradictions or discrepancies among the multiple "selves" can be tolerated under specific conditions. However, these discrepancies among the "selves" must be resolved when they threaten to expose the individual. The discrepancies between the visually impaired person's personal attributes, aspirations, evaluations, standards, and/or values and his significant others' defining attributes, expectations, evaluations, standards, and/or values can be dealt with in one of seven ways: unilateral revision, mutual revision, suppressing the facts, restructuring the situation, selective scanning, distorting the facts, or escape. In response to devaluating stimuli, a person may employ one of a number of defense mechanisms.

Since mental health is associated with self-esteem, characteristics of high and low self-esteem were provided as guidelines for parents and professionals. The sources of self-esteem presented in this unit are the reflections from others, the determination of competence, and the successful management of conflicts and discrepancies.

SECTION III
ADJUSTING WITH BLINDNESS

Chapter 7

THE ADJUSTING PROCESS

ection I provided an introduction to blindness, describing some of the characteristics inherent in the condition of blindness and some of the psychosocial dynamics resulting from blindness. In Section II, two models for the development of self-esteem were applied to persons with visual impairments together with methods for resolving discrepancies for the maintenance of that self-esteem. This section contains a description of the way in which people adjust to a severe crisis or trauma (e.g. either the first recognition of the social stigma of blindness or the onset of blindness) and the restoration of some equilibrium in one's self-concept and self-esteem.

An individual's self-concept and self-esteem are determiners of and responsive to the adjusting process. Hamachek (1971) stated that "The voluminous literature related to the idea of the self and self-concept leaves little doubt but that mental health and personal adjustment depends deeply on each individual's basic feelings of personal adequacy" (p. 225). Anything that interferes with a person's feeling of adequacy, therefore, threatens his personal adjustment and mental health and may result in revisions of the self-concept and self-esteem. At the same time, one's self-concept and self-esteem help to determine the manner of adjusting to the threat of interference. "Self-concept is the person's total appraisal of his appearance, background and origins, abilities and resources, attitudes and feelings which culminate as a directing force in behavior" (LaBenne and Greene,

1969, p. 10). Thus, self-concept and self-esteem are the cause and the effect of the quality of personal adjustment.

Adjusting to the physical or social traumas of blindness is, fundamentally, no different from adjusting to any significant crisis, change, or loss (Bauman, 1954a; Giarratana-Oehler, 1976; Schulz, 1980; Severson, 1953). The title "Adjusting with Blindness" implies the universal process of adjusting to life's demands that are common to all, but with the additional stress of blindness. To one degree or another, divorce, being fired, acquired deafness, loss of a favorite pet, failure in school, severe illness, all require a similar process of adjustment. For purposes of this book, the application of the adjusting model will be confined to the physical and social traumas of visual impairments.

THE MEANING OF ADJUSTMENT

According to Arkoff (1968) the adjusting process is "a person's interaction with his environment, . . . the reconciliation of personal and environmental demands. . . . To be well adjusted, we must adjust well and adjust continually" (pp. 4, 11). Personal and environmental demands change from situation to situation and from time to time. The desirable or valued personal qualities or patterns of behavior may serve a person well in one setting but not in another. Characteristics of good adjustment include "self-insight (knowledge of oneself), self-identity (sharp and stable image of oneself), self-acceptance (a positive image of oneself), self-esteem (a pride in oneself), and self-disclosure (a willingness to let oneself be known to others)" (Arkoff, 1968, p. 17).

Severson (1953) suggested that when working with the adjustment needs of blind persons, professionals would do well to focus on the adjustment needs common to everybody.

Every "adjusted" person should: 1. Have a basic self-respect, 2. Have the ability to see things from the point of view of other people, 3. Know how to use and how to accept authority, 4. Be able to work with persistence toward realistic goals, 5. Have mental alertness and understanding, 6. Have vitality and physical health, and 7. Have as part of himself the ordinary standards of integrity, loyalty, sociability and other important values of his society. (p. 81)

From another perspective, the adjusting process has been described as "learning to accept the reality of a condition and then finding suitable ways to live with that condition" (Acton, 1976, p. 149). When applying this principle to a specific blind person, some questions about whose "reality" and whose judgments of "suitability" begin to arise. "Does adjustment to blindness mean coming to terms with being blind in a sighted world and acting in a way expected of the stereotyped blind, or does it mean trying as far as possible to act as a normal sighted person?" (Delafield, 1976, p. 65). Healthy adjusting requires the discernment of knowing when to appropriate behavior standards and values common to all, whether blind or sighted ("to act as a normal sighted person") and when to appropriate individualized behavior standards and values that are tailored to the individual's personal attributes and characteristics (willingness to use adaptive aids and techniques). In the final analysis, "It is necessary for any blind person to feel he is an integral part of society, that he truly *belongs* to it, is *accepted* by it, and that it is possible to *contribute* to it" (Routh, 1970, p. 48).

The fact that there is no special psychology of blindness, no unique personality of the blind, has been discussed in Chapter 3. However, with respect to acquired blindness, there is disagreement among the professionals as to the impact of blindness on the self. Some argue that good adjustment requires a person to "die" as a sighted self and to be "reborn" as a blind person (Blank, 1957; Carroll, 1961; Cholden, 1958). This implies a new self and a new life.

First, we must realize that those of our clients we call the acquired blind don't only lose something; they acquire something. They add something unto themselves; they add blindness. Such a person lives in a different world, internally and externally, personally and socially. . . . He adds, however, the new concept unto himself of being a different kind of person from all other people and the kind of person he was before. To him, rehabilitation means the reorganization or the bridging of the gap between the old self he was and the new self he must become. This is what rehabilitation is, and it must be done first. The mechanics of life must be attended to: first, the walking, the reading, the earning and the eating; second, his place in the society of man, for now he has a new and unique position; and third, the ways of personal fulfillment—the ways he finds satisfaction and finds his own enrichment.

Rehabilitation, then is a total reconstitution of the being to someone different from the previous being, in preparation for a different life. (Cholden, 1958, p. 110)

The other point of view, and the one preferred by this author, is represented by Wright (1960). "It may be that more often than even wishful thinking would allow man absorbs the fact of a disability in such a way as to keep the major outlines of himself as a person intact. There is good reason to believe that the kind of person one is as differentiated in the self-concept has a stability that resists a general overhaul" (p. 156). This does not preclude the possibility that in some instances blindness does precipitate a complete overhaul of the self. Yet, as a general rule, the fact and implications of blindness can be internalized both intellectually and emotionally into one's personal attributes by modifying some and eliminating others. Nonetheless, the majority of personal attributes remain intact without any need of revision and so preserve the essential nature of the self-concept. (For further discussion of personal attributes, and the process by which they are modified, see Chapters 4, 5 and 6.)

The adjusting process does mean eliminating or extinguishing patterns of behavior that represent exclusively visually oriented standards and values: holding a print hymnbook in church, "looking" at the scenery through the window. It does require a period of time for a person with acquired blindness to make this transition to the point that lack of vision is a natural and integral part of the self and that corresponding behavior is automatic and appropriate. At the same time, blindness must be kept in proper perspective. The individual sees himself first of all as a person and then as a person with many attributes and characteristics, one of which happens to be blindness, rather than seeing himself either as a *blind* person or as a sighted person who doesn't "see so well."

Severson (1953) observed that there are only three adjustments that need to be made solely as a result of the loss of sight itself: "1. The problem of accepting loss of sight in as matter-of-fact a way as possible and so freeing himself from the bitterness, the resentment, the self-pity and the feeling of isolation. . . . 2. The task of acquiring specialized skills. . . . 3. The problem of knowing how to deal with the attitudes and actions of sighted people towards blind people" (p. 81). Some professionals tend to focus on the first of these adjustments. "These psychological problems of blindness invariably have at their core the attitude of the patient toward his affliction" (Cholden, 1958, p. 17). Others tend to stress the development of adaptive aids and techniques. Still others tend to concentrate their efforts on dealing with the attitudes of others. It is "not the nature of the disability, but the reaction of other people to the disability that is important in adjustment" (Delafield, 1976, p. 65). In the final analysis the adjusting process, to be effective, requires a balanced approach to all three issues.

QUALITATIVE ADJUSTMENT

The adjustment of an individual to his visual loss can be seen in the feelings, attitudes, and emotional reactions he demonstrates to three basic questions: "1. How do you look at yourself? (Self-evaluation), 2. How do you look at the other fellow? (His peer group), 3. How do you look at your blindness?" (Routh, 1970, p. 19). A fourth question would reveal additional clues, "How do others look at you and your blindness?" The answers to these four questions are indicators of the nature and quality of a person's current adjustment status, whether healthy, mediocre, or poor.

Many investigators have studied, either directly or indirectly, the adjustment of the visually impaired (they include Bauman, 1954a, 1959, 1964; Cowen et al., 1961; Emerson, 1981; Fitting, 1954; Kirtley, 1975; Lambert et al., 1981; Lukoff and Whiteman, 1970; Miller, 1970; Sommers, 1944; Thume and Murphree, 1961). The following list of characteristics of good and poor adjustment summarizes the observations found in the literature. There is no significance to the order. They represent generalizations drawn primarily from middle-class America, and thus are subject to frequent exceptions. Simply possessing one or two of the characteristics does not necessarily categorize an individual's adjustment, nor does a person in one category have to exhibit all qualities listed.

1. Some characteristics of the visually impaired who are better adjusted:

- Demonstrate psychological stablity.
- Tend to be more intelligent.
- Have a realistic emotional acceptance of blindness.
- Favor independence and tend to be self-directed.
- Have good interpersonal skills.
- Are appropriately assertive.
- Are relatively free of suspicion of others.
- Enjoy and participate in recreational activities.
- Tend to be more educated and have more adjustment training.
- Use adapted aids and techniques without reservation.
- Have a healthy self-acceptance and self-respect.
- Maintain a sense of social integrity.
- Demonstrate independent mobility and adequate daily living skills.
- Acknowledge their kinship with the blind community but not as the sole source of their identity.
- Have family members who show realistic acceptance and understanding of blindness.

2. Some characteristics of the visually impaired who are more poorly adjusted:

- Maintain an unrealistic hope for restoration of sight.
- Tend to be more passive and lethargic.
- Tend toward use of denial mechanisms.
- Demonstrate apathy, withdrawal, and isolation.
- Indulge in self-pity and prolonged depression.
- Are anxious about the future.
- Are preoccupied with doing "something wrong."

- Have low expectations and a poor image of blind persons and are convinced that blindness by itself imputes an inferiority status.
- Believe that blindness is a punishment for sin.
- Strive to meet others' expectations and standards.
- Have families who were/are more overprotective, who react irrationally and adversely to blindness.

Bauman (1964) compared the adjustment of blind adolescents with that of blind adults. She concluded that the adults were more retiring socially, more likely to spend time worrying and "feeling blue," and more likely to react passively to their problems. The students, on the other hand, showed more irritation and suspicion, expressed more of the feeling that they did not deserve their troubles, were more concerned about doing something wrong, were more likely to feel left out of things, and were more likely to fight back. When comparing the anxiety level of ninth and tenth grade blind students with eleventh and twelfth graders, Miller (1970) reported that the older blind students had more anxiety, centering around the areas of social competence, personal appearance, and adjustment to blindness.

Several studies have attempted to compare the self-concept and adjustment of visually impaired children and youth with their sighted peers. Most researchers found no significant difference between the two groups (Coker, 1979; Cowen et al., 1961; Head, 1979; Jervis, 1959; Schindele, 1974; Sommers, 1944). However, Meighan (1971) reported that visually impaired adolescents had significantly more negative self-concepts than did the sighted norm group.

MODELS OF ADJUSTING WITH BLINDNESS

In order to accomplish anything, it is necessary to bring influence to bear upon both the individual and his social world. There are two general directions for attacking such a problem, either to adjust the individual to his environment, or to rearrange the environment so that it ceases to be a difficulty to the individual. It is quite obvious that the latter program is not only inadvisable, but also impossible. However, it is the attack that nearly every frustrated, maladjusted person futilely attempts.

The other alternative is to adjust the individual to his environment as it is. This process can be divided into two major therapeutic programs; first, to redefine the self-regarding attitude of the individual himself; second, to redefine the environmental situation to the individual in terms of the former revised definition of the self. With this sort of clinical and therapeutic picture, it becomes obvious that most of the responsibility for readjustment falls upon the individual himself. (Cutsforth, 1950, p. 186)

Specific disciplines and special interest groups each seem to have their own approach to the resolution of the adjustment problem. The medical model stresses the procedures to restore or correct the anatomical, physiological, and neurological functions of the body, including the function of seeing. The political activists address the problems through their legislative model. The religious domain includes both those who interpret the problem as atoning for sin and those who would heal by the exercise of sufficient faith. The psychological or psychiatric model is concerned primarily with the treatment of neurotic or psychotic maladaptive reactions. The environmentalists attack the problem by attempting to remove the architectural, attitudinal, communication, and transportation barriers in the physical and social environment. In the vocational model, the goal of adjustment is defined in terms of employment. Finally, there are those who focus on education and adaptive training as the key to adjusting with blindness.

The personal adjustment model presented in this section focuses on self-acceptance and self-esteem. It does not seek to minimize or ignore the essential contributions to be made by medical, political, religious, vocational, or educational personnel. Rather, it assumes that these other needs are being or have been met. However, it does not assume that there is necessarily a neurotic or psychotic maladaptive reaction to blindness that must be remediated. As stated earlier, it views adjusting with blindness as a normal process of accommodating to life's many traumas and crises.

Before further developing the personal adjusting model in this unit, it would be helpful to review the contributions of other authors. They are presented in chronological order without extensive description or analysis. The earliest author to be mentioned is Cholden (1958). When working with recently blinded individuals, he observed shock and frequently depression before recovery was possible.

The "dynamics of readjustment" to the onset of blindness were presented by Dover (1959). He described the characteristic reactions as follows:

1. Isolation: withdrawal, blandness, lethargy, shock, disintegration.
2. Depression: low self-esteem, and low frustration tolerance, extreme variability as to intensity.
3. Projection and Denial: blaming others, maintaining hope for recovery.
4. Integration: incorporates blindness into concept of self, realistic management of daily living demands.
5. Mobilization: personal and outside resources, enriched functioning at every level.

Although Cohn (1961, pp. 16-18) was not specifically addressing blindness, her stages of adjustment to a physical disability can be appropriately applied to adjusting to blindness. The inclusion of a "defensive stage" is unique to Cohn. She included the "conditions for change" for each stage. Her stages follow:

1. Shock: "This isn't me." Incompatibility between physical situation and mental picture, possible inappropriate verbal behavior.
   Conditions for change: tests reality, no longer able to function as before.
2. Expectancy of recovery: "I'm sick, but I'll get well." Supercedes all other goals, a prerequisite to the attainment of other goals.
   Conditions for change; return to normal living environment, further testing of reality.
3. Mourning: "All is lost." Feel that worthwhile goals are unattainable, suicidal thoughts, self-pity, possible resignation to "fate."
   Conditions for change: push back and clarify the barrier,

achieve an easily attainable goal.
4. Defensive stage: "I'll go on in spite of it."
   A. Healthy: begins coping, learns to function, some goals still blocked.
      Conditions for change: relinquishing "body whole" value, learn other ways to satisfy needs.
   B. Neurotic: deny any barrier exists, marked use of defense mechanisms, attempt to convince others he is well adjusted.
5. Adjustment: "It's different, but not bad." Disability internalized as one of many characteristics, psychologically normal, able to satisfy needs appropriately, feels he is an adequate person, feels he can be right with God, and is not being punished for his sin.

Using stages similar to Cholden's, Riffenbaugh (1967) presented "states of mental reaction" following the onset of blindness. He discussed three reactions:
1. Shock: immobility, withdrawal, lasts a few days or a few weeks.
2. Depression: self-pity, hopelessness, recriminations, suicidal thoughts, mourning, blames doctors.
3. Adjustment: accepts unpleasant reality, learns new measures to meet life's demands.

Kübler-Ross (1969) is well-known for her study of the various stages involved in adjusting to terminal illness. Although a person with a visual loss is not terminally ill, there are some similarities in the grieving process. She described the stages as follows:
1. Denial and isolation: buffer after experiencing shocking news, temporary defense.
2. Anger: rage, envy, resentment.
3. Bargaining; bargains with God for extension of life.
4. Depression: sense of loss, past and impending.
5. Acceptance: struggle is over, peace with oneself.

An important distinction needs to be made regarding the last stage. The acceptance in this model is the acceptance of death, in contrast to the acceptance in other models in this chapter, the acceptance of the possibilities of life.

Fitzgerald (1970) reported on his work in London with sixty-six individuals between twenty-one and sixty-five years of age who had been registered as blind for less than a year. With the exception of those who had prepared for the trauma of blindness, all the subjects experienced the following sequential, yet overlapping, phases.
1. Disbelief: initial absolute disbelief.
2. Protest: resistance to assistance, training, and use of aids.
3. Depression: suicidal ideation and anxiety, can last days, weeks, or months.
4. Recovery.

Hicks (1979) described the phases of grief, the psychological reaction to loss of sight.

> Grief is the psychological reaction to loss—the gradual process of realisation of the fact and implications of a major loss or change, . . . a dynamically unfolding process, not a fixed state of depression. Its phases and features appear, disappear and reappear, or may be apparently absent. Grief must be worked through to resolution. It cannot be avoided, only postponed, and it cannot be rushed. (Hicks, 1979, p. 170)

The uniqueness of her model is that it begins prior to the actual onset of loss. The phases follow:
1. Preloss: previous personality, previous capacity for stress management, previous overall adjustment.
2. Anticipation: shift from fear and suspicion of impending loss to acknowledge probability.
3. Awareness or confrontation: confirmation, confrontation with reality.
4. Initial reactions: shock, disbelief, denial, anger, guilt, despair.
5. The gradual process of realization: denial, depression, acceptance of the reality.
6. Reorganization, relearning: a turning point, mastery of self-sufficiency acts, increased self-esteem.
7. Resolution: full acceptance, acquired new behaviors, extinguishing nonadaptive behaviors.

There are many other considerations germane to the

adjusting process that are discussed in the literature. Moos and Tsu (1977) described some adaptive tasks that are undertaken by persons in response to a severe illness, but they are equally applicable to people's responses to a visual loss. They are dealt with more simultaneously than sequentially. The adaptive tasks include dealing with pain (physical or psychological) and incapacity, dealing with the hospital environment and treatment, developing adequate relationships with professional staff, preserving a reasonable emotional balance, preserving satisfactory self-image, preserving relationships with family and friends, and preparing for an uncertain future. Other aspects of adjusting with blindness, presented by Giarratana-Oehler (1976), are grieving, reevaluation, independence-dependence conflict, stigma, communication without visual cues, and identity integration.

Many of these adaptive tasks and aspects of the adjusting process will be further elaborated upon in the subsequent chapters of this section. Many of these models share some of the phases or describe phases that are similar. Parts of the model presented in the next chapter also bear some resemblance to one or another of these models. The resultant model represents an integration of the author's reading and research. In the next chapter the phases of adjusting with blindness will follow this sequence:

1. trauma, physical or social;
2. shock and denial;
3. mourning and withdrawal;
4. succumbing and depression;
5. reassessment and reaffirmation;
6. coping and mobilization;
7. self-acceptance and self-esteem.

Since adjusting with blindness is adjusting to life's internal and external demands, it is dynamic and continuous rather than static and fixed (Giarratana-Oehler, 1976). Although the adjusting models reviewed tended to be restricted to the onset of blindness, the concept of adjusting with blindness also permits its application to traumas or crises resulting from experiencing the social stigma of blindness (Delafield, 1976). Adjusting with blindness is not hierarchical, that is, each phase need not be fully accomplished before moving on to the next. Rather, the model is sequential, with people usually experiencing each phase only partially, one at a time, to be revisited and experienced more fully during subsequent encounters (Dover, 1959). The phases are not sharply differentiated, but tend to overlap (Fitzgerald, 1970).

The intensity and duration of each phase varies a great deal from person to person (Dover, 1959). A person can start through the adjusting phases and then stop at a particular phase for a long time or even remain there the rest of his life (Cohn, 1961). Every time a blind person meets a new trauma or a new psychological situation, or discovers a new implication of blindness, he is vulnerable to cycling back through some or all of the adjusting phases (Giarratana-Oehler, 1976; Hicks, 1979). Early preparation for the trauma eliminates much of the later stress and anxiety and minimizes the intensity of subsequent phases (Blank, 1957; Fitzgerald, 1970; Hicks, 1979). A blind person cannot be forced through these phases to hasten the adjusting process but must be allowed to give full expression of his emotions at each phase (Hicks, 1979).

Adjusting with blindness is highly individualistic within the limits of the sequential phases. Both children and adults, both congenitally and adventitiously blind persons experience these phases in one form or another. Even parents or spouses experience a similar adjusting sequence. Other factors that impact upon the adjusting process will be discussed in Chapter 9.

SUMMARY

Self-concept and self-esteem are determiners of and responsive to one's personal adjustment. Adjustment is the reconciliation of personal and environmental demands, a dynamic process that continues throughout life. Adjusting with blindness is adjusting to life with the added stress of blindness. Characteristics of better and more poorly adjusted blind persons were summarized from the literature. Different adjustment models were reviewed together with some of the dynamic qualities of the process.

Chapter 8

SEQUENTIAL MODEL OF ADJUSTING WITH BLINDNESS

The sequential model of adjusting with blindness is a theoretical construct. It is built on the premise that adjusting with blindness follows the same pattern as that of adjusting to any of life's many traumas or crises. Adjusting with blindness is adjusting to life with the additional stress of blindness.

The model of adjusting with blindness is composed of phases that are sequential, rather than hierarchical. To one degree or another, individuals reacting to the physical or social trauma of blindness experience, if only partially, the phases in the order given. The phases tend to overlap without any sharp distinction between one phase and the next. The model is a dynamic, fluid, continuous process without a fixed final "adjustment" at the end. A person may cycle back through some or all of the phases every time he encounters an unfamiliar situation or unresolved discrepancy. An overview of this model was presented in Chapter 3 and is summarized in Figure 14 at the conclusion of this chapter.

A description of each of the adjusting phases is followed by a discussion of the potential role of the professional. The term professional is used to refer to anyone working with blind persons, such as a special education teacher, rehabilitation personnel, social worker, psychologist, or medical personnel. It is assumed that the professional has resolved his own attitudes toward blindness (see discussion on attitudes in Chapter 3) and has analyzed his own value priorities for their potential impact on the blind person he serves (see discussion on values in Chapter 5). This is not an exhaustive manual, but suggested guidelines. Since the phases are overlapping and indistinct, the role of the professional also overlaps from one phase to the next. Suggestions made for one phase may be equally applicable for the previous or subsequent phase.

PHASE ONE: TRAUMA, PHYSICAL OR SOCIAL

"What hit me?"

A trauma is a fact, condition, or circumstance, the awareness of which brings about severe discomfort, turmoil, and anxiety. It is a crisis precipitated by the consciousness of a significant irreconciled discrepancy either intra- or interpersonal (as discussed in Chapters 4, 5 and 6). The trauma introduces an overwhelming threat to the self and the self-concept, upsetting a person's equilibrium and endangering his sense of adequacy.

Initial Trauma for Adventitiously Blind

The sudden and unexpected onset of blindness can be very traumatic, particularly for an individual who is extremely visually oriented in his vocational or avocational interests. The trauma may be compounded by a person's preblindness attitudes toward blindness that are stereotypically negative and devaluating (see Chapters 3 and 9). A trauma for one person becomes a trauma for the significant other close to him (spouse, parent, sibling, or friend). Experiencing retinal detachment was traumatic not only for Sperber, but also for his wife.

> [His reaction] There was a blurring. . . . There were sparks flying. . . . It was a very frightening experience. I went to an ophthalmologist.
> [Her reaction] Of course he was down and very upset. We were both stunned. We didn't know if we should go to another doctor. We were so green about the whole thing. I was sick and scared at first. (Sperber, 1976, pp. 12-14)

The trauma of blindness does not necessarily produce a violent eruption of emotion. Hocken was visually impaired from birth and for her the loss of the remaining vision was not severely traumatic, although elsewhere in her book she aludes to other traumas of blindness.

> Because of the gradual way I had lost what little sight I ever had, I always considered myself fortunate compared with people who had enjoyed perfect vision and then lost it. Naturally I had all the frustrations of being blind, but I never at any point sat down and thought, Last year I could see and now I can't; I shall never get used to this. What am I going to do? (Hocken, 1977, p. 131)

Frequently, the violent turmoil can be tempered or cushioned by one's previous experiences. For Blackhall, the loss of the sight in the second eye seemed to be a repeat of the first trauma some thirty years previous.

> I was playing golf and was walking down the fairway when I saw two balls ahead of me. . . . I cannot pretend that I was either frightened or shocked or disturbed. I experienced no violent reaction whatever. I felt only a cold calm, a kind of detachment as I realised that something was wrong with my vision.
>
> I was with a feeling that I had lived it all before. (Blackhall, 1962, p. 93)

Occasionally, a person will be told long before the actual onset of blindness that they may be losing their vision. In this case the trauma is not the actual loss, but the knowledge of the impending loss. For Mitchell, the doctor's announcement that she would have only "ten years of useful sight" precipitated a series of reactions.

> No other day in my life stands out quite so clearly or so horribly as the day on which I got that verdict. . . . His manner had kept full realisation at bay until I was out in the street, then it struck with such force as to make it touch and go whether I did not go raving and screaming through the heart of Melbourne. . . .
>
> Then I went to see a friend and did break down very thoroughly. Looking back now I rather wonder she did not have enquiries from the police as to whether someone was not being murdered on her premises, but her understanding, aspirin and a good deal more brandy enabled me to pull myself together. (Mitchell, 1964, p. 13)

The younger the person, the less traumatic, relatively

speaking, is the actual onset of blindness (see Chapter 9). The self-concept of a child is not as well formulated, being still pliable and resiliant. The child's style of life and pattern of behavior are not as well established. The reaction of this eight year old, when his mother shared with him that his sight definitely would not return, illustrates a childlike response and reveals some unsatisfied preblindness needs.

> I clearly remember my immediate reaction to the finality of what Mom said. For years I felt guilty about that reaction and, until recently, would not have dared mention it to anybody. I knew a heavy thing had been dropped on me and knew I should probably start crying or something, but I was overcome by a peculiar thrill. Everybody's going to feel sorry for me now. I'll be everybody's little angel and they'll all pay attention. I'll get a lot of presents. Also I could go out and solemnly drop on my friends this heavy, heavy piece of information. (Hartman and Asbell, 1978, p. 36)

Some parents, with the best of intentions, deliberately shield or protect their child from the knowledge that he has a condition that may result in blindness. The subsequent discrepancies the child experiences, frequently in silence, are confusing and difficult to resolve. Referring to a child experiencing a gradual loss of sight without adequate preparation, Blank (1957) said "Under these circumstances, the realization of blindness can be almost as suddenly traumatic as blindness due to an explosion" (p. 12).

Trauma for Congenitally Blind

> My mother always reacted like this. She never told me that I was different from other children, that I could not see as they could. And she never told me that no one in the family—neither she, my father, nor my brother, Graham—could see properly. So I grew up "seeing" things and people differently, yet not knowing there was a difference. As far as I was concerned, it was the little boys over the road who were strange and unusual, not I. (Hocken, 1977, p. 2)

The congenitally blind child experiences a trauma of a different sort. For him, the realization that others can see, while he cannot, grows gradually through repeated encounters of discrepancies. Burlingham (1979) in her work with blind preschool children suggested "as far as we could observe during the nursery school years, the blind child's discovery that other people possess a faculty which he lacks does not come suddenly. It begins as a puzzle which is solved very gradually in . . . stages" (p. 10).

The following excerpt shows how one mother approached the discovery experience in a straightforward and matter-of-fact manner.

> "Look, Mary Sue [his sighted sister], up at the sky. See the stars."
> Davey put up his hand. "I want to see the stars, too," he said. . . .
> I knew that this was my opportunity, the time I had been seeking for. So I put Mary Sue in Al's arms, and I sat down on the steps beside Davey.
> "Listen, honey," I said, and I turned his face toward me. Then I stopped, and for a second, there were no words to say. But then the words came, and I said them. "Davey, some people in this world can't see things with their eyes. Those people are called blind people. They have to look at things with their fingers, the way you do. Annabel is like that, and you are too."
> "But couldn't I touch the stars?" said Davey, and there was, of course, no loss or sorrow in his voice. He had found that very beautiful things could be seen with his fingers. He was only four years old, and so he did not miss color or light when he had shape and substance.
> "No, honey," I said, . . . "some things in this world are too far away to touch, ever, and the stars are like that. Those things you'll have to learn about by hearing of them. Understand?"
> He nodded his head against my shoulder. (Henderson, 1954, pp. 112-113)

For others, the trauma can be more emotional. The discrepancy between personal aspiration and performance may produce a crisis that requires resolution.

> It was my reading lessons, however, that I remember most vividly. I was seated at a kindergarten table. Miss Cook gave me a chart. It wasn't anything like my sister's school books. There were two alphabets on the chart, one in dots, and one in raised letters like those on Mason jars. . . . She showed me "a" in both systems, and told me to look at the letters until I was sure I would know them whenever I saw them.
> When she began working with the other children I buried my head in my arms and sat for a long time. I had been troubled before but never like this.

"Are you sleepy?" Miss Cook asked. "It's pretty early for a little girl to get up."

"I'm not sleepy."

"You aren't homesick?" she laughed.

"No, ma'am. I want to learn to read like Katherine."

"You are going to read like Katherine," Miss Cook said kindly.

"Katherine holds her book in her hand and looks at it, but I feel the letters with my finger."

"The Line Print looks like your sister's book," Miss Cook suggested, "but when you can't see you learn to read with your fingers. It's ever so much nicer than not being able to read at all."

A single tear escaped and rolled down my cheek. . . .

Reluctantly I began examining my chart again, not pacified but accepting the inevitable, and the inevitable was bittersweet. I had believed that by going to school I would be able to read the printed page. Though I was only five I knew now this would never happen. (Brown, 1958, pp. 18-19)

Another trauma for the congenitally blind child is the first awareness of social stigma, disparaging and derogatory attitudes of others, and imputed inferiority status. This childhood trauma is the first realization that others consider him different in more ways than just lack of sight.

In fact, not until I was five years old did I discover that anyone regarded me as different from other children.

In the candy store across from where we lived, I stood at the counter one day, waiting for my licorice and jelly beans. As the shopkeeper slipped them into the bag, I overheard him whisper to the lady next to me, "Such a pretty child—isn't it terrible she's blind."

I can still feel the blood rush to my face and the sting of embarrassment. I dashed home and into the kitchen where Mama was ironing.

"Mama, Mama," I sobbed, "the candy man said it's terrible to be blind. Is it, Mama, is it?" (Resnick, 1975, p. 15)

The awareness of the social stigma of blindness may result in feelings of shame and worthlessness, lowered self-esteem, and self-rejection.

"Oh, I wouldn't fight you," he sneered.

"Why not?" I bellowed.

"Because, you can't see."

I stood there positively stunned.

"What do you mean?" I said, but there was no longer any anger in my voice. . . . He pressed his advantage.

"You heard me," he said, "you can't see."

"Sure I can," I said.

"Okay—" he laughed—"What do you see way over there?" He pointed into the distance.

"Nothing," I said.

"Well, there's a bird there, stupid," he said.

He repeated the test over and over again until it became clear to me that there was something wrong with me.

"The teacher told us never to fight with you because you can't see," Billy told me. . . .

I hated the teacher for differentiating me; I hated Billy for tormenting me and for feeling so superior because he just happened to see; but most of all, I hated myself because I was different. (Krents, 1972, pp. 46-47)

Subsequent Traumas

Subsequent encounters with trauma are frequent for both adults and children. Trauma may recur when one's self-concept and feelings of adequacy that had been previously established are once again threatened. In some instances subsequent and repeated traumas may be precipitated by the jeers and taunts of peers.

Danny was now faced with a new type of problem: his peers. There is something about fifth grade boys that is vaguely reminiscent of *Lord of the Flies*. He was ridiculed on the playground and called "Retardo" and "Spaz." During lunch hour, his cane was frequently taken from him while a bully holding a thermos cup in one hand and Dan's cane in the other staggered around the playground, pitifully crying, "Spare change for the blind. Spare change for the blind." Objects were deliberately placed in his path so he would trip and fall. (Morgan, 1979, p. 45)

In other instances, the stimuli for the additional traumas surface from within the individual in the form of self-doubt and self-recrimination.

I did not know at that time what I have since learned, that this phase of heavy discouragement is a common experience of most persons struggling to emerge from a disaster—from grief, from losses, from problems of every sort. Just as they are riding the crest of the wave of overcoming their condition, a kind of emotional undertow of doubt, of despair, drags them back almost to the starting point of their endeavor. It takes a stout heart to begin all over again. (McCoy, 1963, p. 93)

Although Russell's autobiographical narrative of summer vacations seldom mentioned blindness, but rather focused on enjoyment of life as a competent person, the following incident does illustrate how a frustrating circumstance can precipitate another cycle through the adjusting process.

What a few days earlier had grieved me to the point of fury was the Customs official's assumption that, being blind, I was obviously ignorant, incompetent, in fact, utterly useless. What enraged me now was the sense that he had been quite right. My son at the helm and in skillful command, my wife in the bow with the butt of an oar fending us off and around minor icebergs—and I, I sat amidships, my value consisting in my ability to rock the boat hard and to bounce heavily, thus helping to smash the heavy sheet of ice under the keel. Furious at my impotence, I raged in silence, the knife of my incapacity turning slowly in my vitals. (Russell, 1973, p. 232)

An individual's age at the time of trauma influences his priority of concerns in response to that trauma (see Chapter 9). Each new stage in life brings with it new concerns and new opportunities for trauma. The child experiences his trauma in concert with his needs at the time. The adolescent's changing needs provide new opportunities for additional trauma.

Certainly it was not until my teens that I really began to think about the grave handicap I was stuck with for life.

Of the questions then to be faced, merely those of pursuing higher education and getting into the right job were alarming enough. They were forcing me to deviate still further from the paths to adulthood which the other members of my family were following. (Edwards, 1962, p. 12)

Similarly, adults are more concerned about employment, raising a family and community involvement, which precipitate their own traumas. The traumas experienced by the elderly blind, whether that blindness is congenital or adventitious, center around diminished hearing, health, stamina, independence, and loss of friends through death. The recently blinded elderly person, along with these diminished resources, must also cope with loss of sight.

Role of the Professional

For the adventitiously blind, the trauma frequently begins in the ophthalmologist's office or hospital when the doctor informs the patient that he is losing or has just lost his sight. (See Chapter 9 for further discussion.) On occasion, another professional or parent may also be involved in the awkward and difficult process of communicating this information. In any case, the disconcerting news must be shared with kind and gentle understanding, with direct and simple frankness, and without pity or condescension. Frequently, the traumatized person has already accumulated enough evidence to suspect that the status of his vision has changed. The person who has lived with his suspicions of blindness for a while is usually ready to resolve his uncertainties.

> That doctor was good medicine for me. Never at any time did he allow the slightest tinge of pity to enter his voice. When I was around him, I felt like a normal person, even when discussing my blindness. My blindness was simply a problem that he was helping me to work out. . . .
> I said, "I want to know just what my chances are of ever seeing again."
> "Do you really want the truth?" he said.
> A cold feeling of dread crept over me, but I assured him that I wanted the real dope.
> "Well," he said, "I don't think you will ever be able to see again."
> There it was—the confirmation of the hunch I had had all along. I had expected to be told just that, and I had thought that it wouldn't bother me much. Little did I know! I had tried to keep myself from hoping too much, but I guess a man doesn't realize how much hope he has until that hope is dashed to the ground.
> I stood there speechless! To save my life, I couldn't have made a sound just then. (Fox, 1946, pp. 88-89)

For the one who has had no hint of impending blindess, a more gradual approach is frequently advisable. Statements of increasing certainty over a period of days might take the form: "We have a suspicion that...", "It is possible that...",

"In all probability you. . .", "There is no doubt that. . .", and
". . . has been confirmed, and there is no possibility of
restoration of vision." Dissonant or discordant information
that is confronted suddenly without adequate preparation
is usually more difficult to assimilate and may result in
some unnecessary side effects.

> Bad piece of timing by the darling doctor in this matter, his only
> mistake as far as I know. He brought it up too soon. I wasn't ready,
> family either, tears theirs that time; one had misunderstood on the
> previous visit, thought there was hope. I knew better but even so
> when I heard him sending me to Dr. Zero the bottom fell out. . . . The
> d.d. should have lied a little, said "Maybe eventually, not certain, we'll
> see." (Clark, 1977, pp. 237-238)

To avoid completely or to postpone indefinitely the inevitable can only lead to confusion and bewilderment. The
avoidance of a topic or the speaking of "unmentionables" in
hushed whispers implies a value judgment that something
is dreadfully bad or wrong. If this inference is absorbed by
the traumatized person, it will make his subsequent adjustment process much more difficult. The perceived taboo
regarding open discussion of a particular topic may result in
fear of the unknown and a tendency to employ maladaptive
defensive behaviors.

> This time he did find out what was wrong and told me: I had a
> disease of the eyes called retinitis pigmentosa, and there was no cure
> for it. He called in another specialist who confirmed this opinion, but I
> was left with the impression that things would get no worse. . . .
> May his reticence not create in the mind of the patient when the
> blow does ultimately fall, a mood something like this? "Surely if the
> truth were not so appalling that they thought I could not face it, I
> would have been told! Surely I would have been told if it had been
> believed that there was any chance of my still making something of my
> life even with this disability." (Mitchell, 1964, pp. 10-12)

While the preceding discussion has focused on the adventitious blind, it is equally applicable to the congenitally
blind and their parents. Parents, too, need gentle yet honest
answers to their questions.

> One letter said, quite bluntly, to save our money and energy for the

education which the child would need. But the bluntness was easier to bear than false hopes that were shattered by a word. (Henderson, 1954, p. 47)

Although not all social traumas can or should be prevented, their intensity can be minimized by appropriate intervention. Sometimes parents and professionals may be able to prepare the blind individual for some of the potential encounters with social stigma. At other times, it may be appropriate to provide some explanations to sighted peers regarding the nature and implications of blindness.

Parents and professionals may not always be able to recognize when the blind individual is experiencing a social trauma and therefore miss the opportunity to provide the needed support. The visually impaired person may be unwilling or unable to share these experiences with the significant other, but nonetheless, he may continue to ponder their meaning and significance.

> Not until I went to Trudy's for tea one day did I really come to know that I was a child apart. The television was on, and I was the only one who had to go right up to the screen to recognize the bluish glow of people and flickering objects. Trudy and her mother were sitting back on the sofa, and I could hear them laughing at the program. They said nothing to me (no doubt because my mother had been to see them) to suggest that my having to be so near the set was strange; nor did they complain that I was getting in the way of their view. But somehow I realized they were not simply following it all by sound as we did at home. That evening I did not even bother to ask my mother for an explanation. (Hocken, 1977, p. 7)

Teachers, rehabilitation personnel, and family members must be sensitive and observant to anticipate events that might potentially precipitate a trauma. If at all possible, the blind person should be prepared for the potential social trauma in order to reduce or minimize its impact. The role of the professional after a social trauma has occurred is to provide support and understanding. Corrective intervention with the blind person, as described later in this chapter, should not be taken until subsequent adjusting phases when he is better able to cope.

PHASE TWO: SHOCK AND DENIAL

"I'm too stunned to feel," "I don't believe it's happening."

Shock and denial or disbelief are usually the first reactions to a major trauma or crisis. Shock is a mental numbness, a kind of psychic anesthesia characterized by immobility, depersonalization, and feelings of detachment and unreality. It can occur at any age, from childhood through adulthood, with varying degrees of intensity. While attending a school for the blind, Brown was stunned to hear the doctor's verdict, which was in sharp contrast to the preceeding classmate's prognosis for possible improvement.

> "This is a different story. The trouble here is in the back of the eye," he said after a pause, "She will never see."
> Although I had never really expected to see, I was stunned by the finality of his verdict. I slipped away to my room and cried for a time. Hope dies hard when it dies quickly; and I had never felt so wretched. (Brown, 1958, p. 38)

In contrast to Brown, who was congenitally blind, Clifton also experienced shock when she lost her sight as a teenager due to a detached retina.

> "Keep up your typing and study Braille," he said quietly as he put his arm around my shoulder and patted me gently. Then there was complete silence.
> I was stunned. This meant I was to be totally and permanently blind. This was the end. . . .
> I don't know how long I had sat there in a stupor when I felt Mother tugging at my arm, trying to arouse me.
> "Come, we'd better go home now," she said.
> I faltered as I got to my feet. Suddenly all life seemed to have left me and I clung desperately to Mother's arm. Until that afternoon I had felt strong and had walked alertly with her and my friends. But things were different now.
> I was blind.
> I felt blind and acted blind. Instead of walking I shuffled as Mother led me out onto Michigan Avenue.
> I asked if there was a cab at the curb.
> "Yes," she replied. "But why a cab?"
> "So we can get home."
> "We came down on the bus."
> "I know, but that was different. Don't you understand? I'm blind."

"We'll go home on the bus," she said firmly, and we did. (Clifton, 1963, pp. 16-17)

Cholden, a psychiatrist who worked with blind patients, described the shock phase:

> During this period, which may last from a few days to a few weeks, he finds himself unable to think or feel. (One patient aptly described this time in terms of feeling "frozen." He felt nothing.) It would seem that his new task is so formidable that he must approach it by retrenching all his energies for a time. He reacts to the feeling of imminent chaos and disintegration by an emergency constriction of his ego.... We can then think of this shock stage as a period of protective emotional anesthesia which is available to the human organism under such stress. (1958, pp. 73-74)

The shock reaction is healthy and normal, for it shields the individual from being suddenly overwhelmed by the full impact of the trauma. As the psychic anesthesia begins to wear off, the individual may still be unwilling or unable to handle the reality of the situation. Initially, the use of some defense mechanisms such as denial, rationalization, and repression (see Chapter 6) is normal and adaptive. Only when their use persists does it become maladaptive (Hicks, 1979). An individual may employ a variety of strategies to protect his psychic equilibrium because he cannot immediately assimilate or integrate the fact and all the resultant implications of a major trauma or crisis (Parkes, 1972). "Depersonalization seems to be an emergency defense against the threat of dissolution of the ego by eruption of overwhelming painful affects. The affects are thereafter allowed to emerge bit by bit so that they can be handled by the ego piecemeal" (Blank, 1957, p. 11).

> The implication of blindness was horrifying. Indeed, the doctor's suggestion produced a sense of shock so profound that a part of my mind seemed to stop functioning, and the terrified thoughts that had scampered through my brain at the first realization of the possibility of my becoming permanently and totally blind were put away into some inner fastness and I refused to let them out.
>
> "He's only trying to frighten me into being a docile patient." I told myself. "He doesn't really mean it." I clung to this rationalization as I followed a nurse down a corridor and into a room where she helped

to undress me. So within a matter of hours I was snatched from a life filled with excitement and action to the monotony of a hospital bed. (Carver, 1961, p. 140)

Denial

Denial is one of the most common psychic defenses employed during the shock phase. There are two forms of denial, either of which can be partial or full (VanderKolk, 1981). The first is a disbelief, a refusal to acknowledge, a rejection of the fact that a trauma has even occurred.

I could not believe that my eyes were "permanently, irreparably, and irrevocably" damaged. I could believe it in my head. . . . But I didn't live in my head, I lived in what Christians call "the heart." . . . It was my heart that refused to accept the verdict. I was denying the truth. It was unpleasant and painful. . . . Surely it was a bad dream and I would awaken. Surely there was a cure out there that would heal my hurt in here.

I could not be healed until I accepted the finality of the facts. (Kemper, 1977, pp. 75-76)

The second is an unrealistic expectation that a miracle from God, a medical procedure, or a new scientific discovery will restore vision. When this persists, "hope for recovery, which is so important a therapeutic tool in all other aspects of medicine, is a major deterrent to adjustment to blindness" (Cholden, 1958, p. 23).

A . . . teacher singled me out for special attention and friendship, taking me for walks and giving me candy. One day he said, "A friend of mine who lost his sight prayed every day to get it back. Sure enough, one morning he woke up and could see a little better; next day, still better; another day, better yet. Just by praying." . . .

So every night, after reading my Bible in Braille, I would add to my string of prayers a plea to see again. . . .

One day another teacher mentioned something that would be required of me next year when I'd be a residential student. I replied, "I won't be here next year." She asked, "Why not?" I said, "My sight will be coming back." She said with annoying firmness, "Your sight's not coming back." "Yes it is," I argued, but she wouldn't budge. (Hartman and Asbell, 1978, pp. 34-35)

Schulz (1980) discussed two consequences of utilizing denial as a form of adjusting. The first consequence is that the individual refuses services and aids that could benefit him. The second is that he is tempted to engage in foolish or dangerous activities that require more vision than he in reality possesses. While driving, James Thurber certainly engaged in an activity dangerous to both his wife and to himself.

> Helen Thurber and I have just returned from dinner at the Elm Tree Inn in Farmington, some twenty miles from our little cot. It was such a trip as few have survived. I lost eight pounds. You see, I can't see at night and this upset all the motorists in the state tonight, for I am blinded by headlights in addition to not being able to see, anyway. It took us two hours to come back, weaving and stumbling, stopping now and then, stopping always for every car that approached, stopping other times just to rest and bow my head on my arms and ask God to witness that this should not be. (Bernstein, 1975, pp. 275-276)

The severity of the shock phase not only varies from person to person but may also vary within the same person from one time to the next. Schulz (1980) identified three factors that help to influence the intensity of the shock. "The severity of the shock experienced by a person is determined to some extent by the significance to him of what he has lost. . . . A second factor that determines the severity of shock may be the suddenness or unexpectedness of the event. . . . Similarly, the degree of visual loss will affect the extent to which the individual feels the shock" (pp. 24-25).

Role of the Professional

Cholden (1958) hypothesized that "the longer the shock state, and/or the greater the number of shock episodes, the more difficult is the person's rehabilitation to blindness" (p.74). This does not imply that the professional should attempt to hasten the individual through the shock and subsequent phases. In fact, any attempt to do so is counterproductive. The role of the professional is simply to make himself available, to provide physical comfort, emotional support, and understanding.

> Either she [a friend] or her sister had met every bus since a mutual friend had telephoned the news at lunch time, and they had, I

gathered, spent most of the afternoon in appalled lamentations. The knowledge of this helped me a little for it showed understanding, and it was understanding and kindness I needed, not any attempt at comfort. In the first shock of any major disaster there is no possibility of comfort, and any attempt at it, any well meaning effort to point out that things might be worse, only causes irritation and increases suffering, particularly when the comforter has no firsthand knowledge of your affliction. That at least has been my experience. It was so now, and for the next few weeks I lived through such a period of fear and horror and misery as I had never envisaged in those moments when I believed I had faced the prospect of blindness. Dominating everything was the sense of being trapped, of not knowing where to turn or how to set about even trying to grapple with the situation. For of that one thing I was quite certain: it had to be grappled with. (Mitchell, 1964, p. 14)

The individual's defenses prevent him from assimilating any more implications of blindness or new information regarding rehabilitation. In the state of stunned numbness, the individual is unable to deal with an analysis of past mistakes, a comparison with other "sufferers," or the "things are going to get better" approach. This is not the time to try to deal with the denials and unrealistic expectations.

For the person experiencing shock, time is probably a more important factor than any direct intervention by a professional. The professional can and should be available to provide support and comfort. However, it is with time that the psychic anesthesia or numbness begins to wear off. Slowly but surely, bit by bit, the individual begins to acquire a general sense of the reality of the situation. It is the confrontation with this reality that stimulates a person to progress further through the subsequent phases of the adjusting process.

The shock itself may be of what might be termed therapeutic value. Complacency is no good beginning for adjustment, which implies the individual's wish to move and to propel himself. Certainly in my case shock itself was of value. It had the effect of making me want to put behind me the false hopes of the immediate past. And though I had no relish for the immediate future, it gave me the impetus to face it. (Chevigny, 1946, p.32)

If the traumatized person begins to use defense mechanisms to avoid honestly facing his situation, the professional will need to confront him gently but persistently with the reality of the trauma. Whether the shock was precipitated by onset of blindness or by an encounter with a social stigma, whether the individual is a child or an adult, any further progress through the adjusting phases depends on the degree to which he is able to comprehend intellectually and to accept emotionally the fact that a trauma has occurred. However, his awareness of the many specific implications of the trauma does not occur until later during the succumbing phase. The intervening phase of mourning is the more immediate reaction to the acknowledgement of the reality of the trauma.

PHASE THREE: MOURNING AND WITHDRAWAL

"Poor me," "No one understands"

When the numbing effects of shock begin to dissipate, one commences to mourn or grieve the loss of something important and valuable (Cohn, 1961; Schulz, 1980; Wright, 1960). The gradual increase in one's awareness of the inescapable reality and the decreasing use of the initial psychic defense behaviors occur simultaneously and are interdependent.

> The outcry of a new-blind person is very like that of a newborn babe—it is filled with protest, outrage, and fear. I too cried out in protest against my fate. I cried out in fright—yes, in self-pity. At first I said, "I cannot believe it," and then I said, "I will not believe it," but finally, fatigued beyond measure, I said, "I suppose I must believe it." And then the hard cold fact of the situation confronted me in its grim reality. A numbing terror fastened itself upon me when I was thus brought to realize that I was doomed to live the rest of my life in complete darkness. There was an agonizing feeling of helplessness and dismay at the thought of going through day after day without eyesight. . . .
> How could I endure the agony of having this part of my life removed, severed, amputated? (McCoy, 1963, p. 20)

Mourning is characterized by self-pity. During this period

of time, one has the feeling that all is lost. The grieving may be for the initial loss of sight or for subsequent further loss of vision. Chevigny described the frustration and self-pity that he felt when first trying to walk after spending three months in bed because of detached retinas.

> You've got to find that bed because your knees are beginning to buckle. But it's hard to ask her [the nurse] for that help, to admit that you're lost. It seems a surrender, a lowering of your pride. And you wonder why it is so difficult to admit that you need her help. . . .
>
> [After getting back in bed] I wept, for perhaps the first time in thirty years. They were tears of frustration, rage, emotional exhaustion, and considerable self-pity. . . . And there was no escaping the realization that this was only the beginning, only the first fifteen minutes of a new lifetime. (Chevigny, 1946, pp. 20-21)

In response to a social trauma, mourning is a feeling of being sad or sorry for a perceived loss of adequacy, self-esteem, equality, belongingness, or control in a vague, global sense.

> All the frustrations and loneliness of adolescence poured out in song after song. . . .
> I wish I was an apple
>   Hanging from a tree;
> I wish I was most anything
>   Except a boy like me. (Krents, 1972, pp. 125-126)

As the psychic anesthesia continues to wear off, the individual may begin to experience a whole host of other emotions: apathy, bitterness, fear, boredom, helplessness, and frustration. Many of these emotions are common to most people with or without blindness. It would be difficult to determine which emotional reaction was due to blindness and which was due to life apart from blindness. Suffice it to say that blindness only serves to exacerbate personality predispositions toward any of these emotional expressions.

Persons who are absorbed in their self-pity are so preoccupied with their own problems and concerns that they find it difficult to be aware of others and their needs. They have a tendency to focus on the visual loss and the problems they perceive surrounding blindness to the exclusion of other more normal and more routine needs. In short, they become egocentric, with a very restricted range of interests and concerns.

> "You know what I think, Andrew?" she said, her voice dry and cool. "I think that all you're ever really concerned about is your goddamn eyes." (Potok, 1980, p. 242)

Withdrawal

Another common phenomenon during the mourning phase is the withdrawal or pulling back from contact with one's physical and/or social environment. Prolonged withdrawal, which can be physical and/or emotional, results in feelings of isolation and loneliness. Temporary withdrawal is a natural consequence of the social or physical trauma of blindness until one can develop new or better adaptive coping skills.

> This anger and soul-searching were but part of the story in those days. There were some other wonderful and gracious events happening to me, too. But the trouble with elephants is that they cannot see the real world clearly; they cannot see the love that is still for them and with them. . . .
>
> All I knew was that this elephant was angry and was not seeing the supportive love of his family, friends, and church. . . .
>
> It did not become real or clear to me until some time later, but even in this time of desperation I was the beneficiary of some powerful help. My children do not love me for my eyes. . . . My friends at church wanted to speak to me, but what was there to say to me? I did not initiate conversation so they ignored what had happened. That made me think they had forgotten and were going on their merry ways. . . . And as for God. . . . "Thy rod, and thy staff they comfort me." There was a rod and a staff there, but I could not grasp them.
>
> An angry elephant alone on an island feels very sorry for himself. (Kemper, 1977, pp. 72-73)

Unfortunately withdrawal can become one's habitual manner of coping with an unbearable reality (Schulz, 1980). Extreme withdrawal and self-imposed isolation are unnatural and unhealthy.

Expressions of hostility and anger are also common during the mourning phase. Hostility may manifest itself as constant irritability or as an occasional sudden outburst. It may be directly attributable to a frustrating situation imposed by blindness or it may be apparently unrelated to anything that has happened (Schulz, 1980).

> I went to my club for lunch, and sat opposite a woman whom I had known slightly for a long time, and who in my opinion had made little use of her life. Her presence filled me with such jealousy because she was keeping her sight while I was losing mine, that I could hardly speak civilly to her. (Mitchell, 1964, p. 13)

Schulz (1980) suggested that "hostility as a reaction to the loss of sight is most likely to be displayed during the early period following the loss. It is during this time that the person is experiencing the greatest stress. . . . If the individual has never resolved the feelings stemming from his loss, the hostility may become an integral part of his personality" (p. 65). Sullivan demonstrated some unresolved hostility as he contemplated the preparation of a speech he was asked to deliver.

> I would tell them of my childhood and pay tribute where it was due to the dedicated people who had helped me. Mostly I would talk in anger.
> I thought of how a child goes to a blind school. . . carrying with him no sense of personal identity, having had little or no contact with other children. . . .
> I reflected on how a blind child is caught, trapped in the web of "blindisms," how he is surrounded by other children with his own handicap and with children who have other problems such as mental deficiency, which not infrequently goes with blindness. . . .
> It was upon the administrators that my anger focused, . . . so convinced that they were doing a great job because they provided good equipment and a beautiful campus. (Sullivan and Gill, 1975, pp. 170-171)

Mourning is a normal, healthy, and necessary reaction to a generalized feeling of a vague, global loss, precipitated by a severe physical or social trauma. Fortunately, a person usually becomes saturated with self-pity, growing sick and tired of feeling sorry for self (Wright, 1960). Occasionally, however, a person will resign himself to the "fate" of his loss and continue to wallow in self-pity and grief for months and even years.

Role of the Professional

During the mourning phase, part of the role of the professional consists of being a good, discerning listener. "For a short time the patient should be allowed to mourn for his dead eyes. After the mourning, he can then slowly proceed in the rehabilitation process" (Cholden, 1958, p. 26). The professional will want to continue to provide physical comfort, emotional support, and understanding. Giving expression to one's sadness can be therapeutic (Riffenburgh, 1967).

> I have already spoken about the poems I wrote in the hospital. If, running through these poems, there was the drumbeat of grief, I like to think that there was also the ringing note of hope for anyone who cares to look for it. On one occasion my wife, who is a very sensitive person, said to me: "Why do you tear your heart out, writing stuff like this?"
>
> "I assure you that I am not tearing out my heart," I replied. "I am tearing the sadness and the pain out of my heart and my heart is the better for it. Once I have formulated it and given it tongue, it is over and done with." (Blackhall, 1962, p. 125)

During this period of mourning and self-pity, the blind individual feels incompetent and inadequate to meet the demands of life. The professional needs to counteract these feelings by providing some easily mastered, practical solutions to personal and social management problems. The new information or skill can serve as convincing evidence that all is not lost, that life is indeed possible as a blind person.

The professional would be well-advised to remember that some blind persons, especially during this mourning phase, resent the well-intentioned encouraging remarks from sighted people. After all, they reason, sighted people cannot possibly know what it is like to be blind.

This is not to suggest that all sighted people are incapable of offering support or understanding nor that all blind people resent all sighted individuals. However, there is a time when the credibility of a message is much stronger coming from another blind person. The professional may want to arrange for a competent blind person to meet with the individual who is mourning. Areas of concern to be discussed with the recently blinded might include some "tricks of the trade" or some quickly and easily learned adaptive techniques. For the socially traumatized, it may simply be to share some practical advice regarding the handling of derogatory and devaluating remarks and actions.

> Of those who have turned to me the largest percentage is, I believe, of persons struggling with fear—fear of what their handicap, no matter what it is, will do to them in their field of work, in their social relations with their fellow men. . . . I always try to point out that what is oppressing them is a twofold fear—fear of the handicap itself, the problem, the loss—and also fear of the emotional torment which usually accompanies these things. I urge them to perceive the difference between the two. (McCoy, 1963, p. 194)

However, the individual is not yet ready for lectures on the need for rehabilitation, for advice about how lucky one is, or for sermons about the many other successful people who happen to be visually impaired. McCoy's effectiveness in counseling with others was due in part to the fact that she herself had worked through similar problems.

> I would not listen to reminders that thousands of others down the centuries had learned to live in the darkness of blindness. . . . I resented being reminded—in what struck me as dour and pious tones—of some of those who had born blindness bravely. . . .
>
> All that had been so close, so ready at hand and—alas—so matter-of-factly accepted, was now far removed, as distant as outer space, if indeed it existed at all.
>
> This sense of removal began to mount to a feeling of exile from everything that had constituted my life as a sighted person. In my new blindness I was dismayed, confused, terrified, for what had happened to me had banished me to an alien world—a strange, unfriendly world, a world that seemed without hope or interest, a world in which from the start I was homesick for my native land, the land of the sighted. (McCoy, 1963, pp. 20-23)

The general atmosphere and schedule of daily routine during this time are critical. Emerson (1981) found that readjustment is more difficult for those continuing to live with others who exhibit predominantly adverse social reactions and attitudes (see Chapter 3). If at all possible, the professional should try to intervene and ameliorate such conditions.

It is beneficial during this mourning phase for the blind person increasingly to redirect his mental energies off himself and onto other activities to impede the withdrawal or isolation. The professional may need to intervene by structuring or providing appropriate activities to occupy the blind individual's time. A busy life tends to take a person's mind off himself and to reduce the time spent in self-pity. The blind person may be unable to plan these activities for himself during the mourning phase. With a little guidance, friends and other acquaintances are frequently in the best position to develop and implement these activities. The pattern of behavior established during the days following the trauma frequently sets the tone for the remainder of the adjusting process.

> Within a few days of my coming home [from four months in the hospital], a friend rang me and invited me to the Rotary Club luncheon. Suddenly, I wanted to hide myself away. I am quite sure that, in a flash, I experienced all the emotions which had made my friend of former years voluntarily inaccessible to the many hands which were eager to reach out to him in tenderness and love. It is now or never, I thought.
>
> "Certainly I will come," I answered, though my heart was in the basement. "It is very good of you to ask me." (Blackhall, 1962, pp. 115-116)

After a period of time the mourning for the global loss gives way to an increasing awareness of the many complications resulting from the trauma. The gentle, persuasive confrontation with the necessity to manage life's demands in a new and different way can be used to assist the individual to move beyond the generalized sense of sadness and mourning to an analysis of the more specific consequences of his new circumstances.

PHASE FOUR: SUCCUMBING AND DEPRESSION

"I can't," "I'm distressed"

Mourning for the global loss is followed by a gradual process of becoming more and more aware of specific implications of that loss.

> You know almost certainly that you will not be able to see, but you do not know much about what goes with it. It may be a long time before you have the full realization of all that it implies. (Pierce, 1944, p. 19)

During the succumbing phase, the traumatized individual itemizes and analyzes the perceived effects of the trauma, whether realistic or not. When the perceived effects go beyond the realistic consequences imposed by blindness, the person is said to be engaging in the "spread" phenomenon (Wright, 1960). Milder forms of depression usually accompany this phase, with many of the same emotions and behavior patterns from the mourning phase continuing: self-pity, lethargy, withdrawal, isolation, loneliness, helplessness, boredom, frustration, anger, and hostility.

> The Anatomy of Affliction—will that do? Or The Afflicted Anatomy. But my dear lady, you're only dealing with a physical disability, sudden and mysterious to be sure, but not very dire as such things go, not likely to be total (as in totaling a car) nor even involving any physical pain, furthermore occurring among those blessings that are so joyously to be counted. "Ghastly deprivation," "hideous handicap" say the letters from friends. I said, "But, Doctor, what you're telling me is to me a lot worse than death." It was no lie. If you're totaled, does it matter if wheels and a fender are still good for scrap? (Clark, 1977, p. 57)

The succumbing phase is characterized by negativism and pessimism. The individual seems to focus only on the negative implications of the trauma, often exaggerating their effects unreasonably. This is the "I can't" phase when the individual concentrates his thoughts on abilities and capacities thought to be lost. All valued goals seem to be blocked; he is unable to perceive any worthwhile attainable goals remaining to him (Cohn, 1961).

> "I'm just a goddamned blind kid," I whined. "I thought I could fight my way out of the snake pit of blindness, but now I know that I can't. I'm gonna have to spend the rest of my life weaving baskets or whatever. Who the hell said I could make it in the sighted world? You know damned well I can't. You know I haven't got a chance. Why was I born blind? Go on, answer that one. It'd been better if I'd been born Mongolian or a village idiot. Then I wouldn't have to think. I wouldn't have ambition. They could have given me a tin mug and a busy street

corner and I'd have been reasonably happy. It's people like you who've made my life a hell. You've tried to make me reach for the impossible. I'm blind, don't you understand that, Bill? I'm blind! Blind! Blind!" (Sullivan and Gill, 1975, p. 94)

The introspection of the succumbing phase intensifies a person's feelings of inadequacy and incompetence and thus reinforces his low self-esteem. The negativism and pessimism regarding current abilities and potential goals can be experienced both by the congenitally blind, as illustrated above by Sullivan, and by the recently blinded, as illustrated by Kemper.

Listening to one of my oral tirades over some trivial matter, seven-year-old Ginny asked her mother, "Why is Daddy so angry?" Stupid people! Could they not understand that I was angry not because of them or the trivial instance which had brought on the flare-up? Of course they could not. They could not because the cause was in me. I looked the same as I always did, and for the most part I acted the same as I always did. There was nothing external that was different from what I always had been. But inside my head, behind those wounded eyes, an elephant raged. I cannot do it, he bellowed. I'll never make it. (Kemper, 1977, p. 71)

According to Wright (1974), the characteristics of succumbing are as follows:

1. Emphasis on what the person *can't do*.
2. Little weight is given to the areas of life in which the person can participate.
3. The person is seen as *passive*, as beaten down by difficulties.
4. The person's accomplishments are minimized by highlighting their shortcomings, usually in terms of "normal" standards.
5. The negative aspects of the person's life, such as the pain that is suffered or difficulties that exist, are kept in the focus of the person's life. They are emphasized and exaggerated and even seem to usurp all of life (spread).
6. The disability represents such an unadjustable state that one must try to hide and deny it. Some kind of adjustment is possible only by acting as if it doesn't exist. Resignation is the only other alternative.
7. Whether or not the person is able to hide his disability, he is pitied. (p. 115)

Whether blind or not, the person who is always saying "I

can't" to everything, who feels that all goals are blocked, who feels there is nothing left that is worthwhile, is certainly miserable and to be pitied.

"Losses"

Much of the literature, both popular and professional, focuses on the perceived succumbing aspects of blindness at the expense of the other phases of the adjusting process. For example, Carroll (1961) expounded upon twenty "losses" that he had observed in recently blinded adults, many of whom were war-blinded veterans. Yet, to place too little emphasis on the succumbing phase is as inappropriate and foolish as emphasizing it too much. For most, blindness is more than a mere inconvenience and must be confronted in its true significance.

The perceived negative implications of blindness are highly individualistic. The "losses" a person identifies are dependent upon his activities, aspirations, standards, values, and relationships. Because of the tremendous variability, the following discussion of the perceived negative consequences of blindness is not intended to be exhaustive. The illustrations used are only a small representative sample taken from biographies and autobiographies. It must be remembered that, during the succumbing phase, the "losses" described may not be very realistic or even directly attributable to blindness; they are simply personalized perceptions.

Some of the comments center around the perceived loss of self-esteem and self-worth and loss of the sense of adequacy, of being in control of oneself and one's environment. Emerson (1981) reported that reactions to loss of vision among members of her low vision support group were characterized by a sharp loss of self-esteem, a certainty that they were discredited, and the feeling that they were neither attractive nor able to function normally.

> But that night after the lights were out and the ward was quiet, it was a different matter. I pray God I never have to live through another night like that one. What would I do, what could I do to make a living?

How could I raise my son? What was it going to be like never to see the faces of my loved ones again? (Fox, 1946, p. 91)

Observations of the newly blind frequently express the loss of the ability to manage their own activities of daily living. Feelings of regression to infantile dependency are common until suitable adaptive skills are mastered.

I could easily reach the bedside table, my fingers found the wireless and, when I wanted it, the spouted cup with the orange juice. But the moment I left my bed, the weight of helplessness came crashing down on me. Only now did I appreciate what it meant when I could see a little. While a tiny bit of light still penetrated my pupil, I could move about a little, relying on the outlines of people and objects, but now I was entirely defenseless, at the mercy of my environment. I became an infant who has to be fed and bathed, because I could no longer do anything for myself.

I became a giant baby in a huge grandfather chair. (Vajda, 1974, p. 142)

Other comments tend to focus on the perceived loss of sensory stimulation or on the more restricted sources for mental stimulation. There are some who, without adequate training or retraining, are frustrated from a sense of boredom, of time weighing heavily. The more restricted sensory stimulation reduces the number of choices available to him, choices of activities, of alternative courses of action.

What is more serious is my fear that the quality of my work has suffered, for as I had foreseen would be the case, loss of sight has limited my sources of inspiration. My imagination is no longer stimulated into action by something I have seen, as so often happened in the past. . . .

The blind man's field of study is limited by his disability, for it is liable to restrict his movements and to make him lose the initiative in intercourse, thus lessening the number of his social contacts. . . .

He has a good chance of noting changes in colloquial speech, but he can't detect changes in clothes, furnishing or gadgets. . . .

Another form of figures from direct contact with which the blind man is debarred is telephone numbers. . . . The blind man cannot read correspondence, . . . the whole of a menu. (Mitchell, 1964, pp. 32-52)

Some blind individuals describe the succumbing in terms of a loss of personal freedom or independence. The areas of life vulnerable to this scrutiny vary from one individual to another: economic/employment, travel/driving, recreation.

> Intellectual freedom is the only freedom I have today, for blindness has destroyed my physical freedom. (Bretz, 1940, p. 28)

> The thing that upset Al more than losing his sight was losing the ability to play tennis and Ping Pong. (Sperber, 1976, p. 14)

The perceived loss is frequently discussed in terms of difficulties in interpersonal relationships. Schulz (1980) felt that some of the dilemma stems from a basic fear of abandonment, a fear that a meaningful relationship will be terminated. Resentment and bitterness develop around the apparent dependency needs of the blind person. Much of the stress in interpersonal relationships is rooted in the devaluating and derogatory attitudes held about blindness. One's feeling of sexuality are unnecessarily victimized and frequently stunted.

> [When on vacation from the residential school] But even here, amid the chink and clatter of the holiday dinner, I was still in isolation. Though I was in that other world, I was not of it. My family and their friends accepted me completely, of course, but I had no real friends my own age. I must have understood something of my loneliness because, when I did make my first friends, I was overwhelmed with joy. (Russell, 1962, p. 76)

Depression

Dobson (1975) has described depression and emotional apathy as the condition of "the D's": "despair, discouragement, disinterest, distress, despondency and disenchantment with circumstances as they are" (p. 15). Depression, he said, is a common and recurring fact of life. It is not surprising, then, to find Jourard (1963) and Hicks (1979) commenting that depression is a natural and normal response when adjusting to a severe trauma. It may be in response to the "losses" already analyzed, or it may be in response to some anticipated "losses" yet to be exposed.

VanderKolk (1981) stated that "the disagreeable change in self may result in many psychological symptoms: withdrawal, anger, self-pity, self-hate, suicidal thoughts, feelings of hopelessness, and bitterness. The client's depression will vary in intensity over a period of time. With support from rehabilitation workers, family, and friends, the depressive states become less intense and less frequent" (p. 143).

> Then one day a clear certainty about my situation took possession of me—the certainty that I was helpless, powerless, finished. I was pinned beneath the debris of the calamity which had fallen upon me, debris as pressing, as suffocating as any resulting from an earthquake or a hurricane. I knew there was no strength in me to lift any part of this mass. Can anyone come to my rescue, I wondered. Can anyone reach me—can anyone even know the extent of my plight? It is unlikely.
>
> The sad and sodden part was that suddenly, and for the first time in my life, I had no desire to make any effort to help myself. Nothing was worth the doing, nothing worth a struggle in this dead-end existence. I sank back, surrendering myself to "make my bed in Hell," as the Psalmist puts it. It does not matter, I sighed, and let myself sink slowly down into the gloom—interested in nothing, expecting nothing. (McCoy, 1963, p. 26)

The fact that the emotions experienced during the succumbing phase resemble those of a reactive depression has been the source of some confusion. "As the newly blinded patient begins to experience emotions again, what he feels, and the way he reacts, seems similar in all respects to what is often called a 'reactive depression.' We see the usual self-recriminations, feelings of hopelessness, self-pity, lack of confidence in meeting problems, suicidal thoughts and psychomotor retardation" (Cholden, 1958, p. 75). Rather than being a psychiatric disorder, temporary depression is a normal, therapeutic phase of the adjusting process. "Awareness that this depression is a mourning reaction rather than a psychiatric disorder requiring treatment is essential if we are to avoid . . . attempts to force the patient to turn his psychic energies to the problems of the external world before he has accomplished the inner work of mourning" (Blank, 1957, p. 12).

The therapeutic value of depression was emphasized by Hicks 1979) when she commented that depression is—

> potentially healing. It can lower responsiveness and act as a protective screen; it can act as a cut-out when basic survival is threatened so that adaptation can come later; it can have a

cathartic effect of releasing pent-up emotional tension by weeping; and it can be thought of as a period of inward diversion of energy while the individual adapts to external traumatic events. (p. 172)

Severe Depression

While some depression of a temporary nature can be considered a normal response to trauma, serious and prolonged depression is not. According to Blank (1957), more serious maladaptive depression expresses itself as a chronic masochistic state, with self-recriminations and bitterness toward the world and God. While individuals are reacting in this way, they will never be able to accept the reality of the trauma, will remain hostile, yet dependent, and will resent the people upon whom they are dependent.

Severe depression is characterized by acute and sustained feelings of despair, despondency, and hopelessness. Despite a sullen, dominating, critical, and hostile attitude, these individuals have an intense need for affection and frequently exhibit a desire for social approval. They are "so overwhelmed by anxiety, depression and shame that they cannot think of constructive ways to fulfill themselves" (Lambert et al., 1981, p. 194). The intensity of the depression is a function of the intensity of the withdrawal pattern established during the mourning phase (Schulz, 1980). Dover (1959) suggested that "reactive depression does not always follow loss of vision. Usually when a person is depressed, there is a history of previous disturbance, particularly of low frustration tolerance to stress situations and a marked feeling of low self-esteem" (p. 335).

Emerson (1981) mentioned several other factors that were associated with prolonged depression in members of her low vision therapy group: (1) loss of vision was accompanied by other losses, such as death of a family member or disease; (2) there was a lack of support from the family; and (3) the impairment was severe when compared with other members of the low vision group.

The state of intense despair, despondency, and hopelessness may lead to suicidal thoughts (Hicks, 1979). Most suicidal thoughts and death wishes soon disappear. Some are verbalized into threats and even less are specifically planned out (Schulz, 1980). Very few result in actual suicide (Fitzgerald, 1970).

> I took two steps forward as I heard a large delivery truck come toward me. One more step and my worries would be over. With one foot raised, I suddenly halted. . . . . I seemed to freeze momentarily, then I drew back quickly. The driver blew his horn, swerved, and just missed me by inches. Then he jammed on the brakes.
>
> My emotional storm quieted as quickly as it had blown up. The screeching brakes told me that the truck had stopped and that the driver probably was coming back toward me. . . . "I'll never do it again, because now I've changed my mind," I told him. (Sheppard, 1956, pp. 43-44)

The state of succumbing, then, can be conceived of as the accumulated barriers that impede or prevent a person from reaching desired goals, and depression is the accompanying emotional reaction. Blocked goals produce frustration and anxiety. If the individual assumes personal responsibility as the causal agent for the barrier, a certain amount of guilt will also accompany the succumbing phase. Focus on the perceived succumbing "losses" elicits pity, condescension, and even contempt from the nonblind. Likewise, prolonged fixation on the "losses" contributes to even more severe depression for the recently traumatized and his significant others.

Role of the Professional

Much of the same approach initiated during the mourning phase will need to be continued. The succumbing person remains in urgent need of emotional support and understanding. Expressions of resentment, frustration, and hostility will still be common. Family members who are providing much of the needed support and understanding will not be able to comprehend, unless prepared, just why they have become targets of the hostility and resentment. The professional needs to interpret the dynamics of the adjusting process to family members and friends.

I had run away from the sources of life that were for me, self-indulgently licking my wounds and playing the part of helpless victim even in my achievements. I wanted to be loved for something I wasn't, an unfortunate victim of circumstance. I could not accept the love that was given me for what I was and not for what I was not. I had made a cage of my problem, and what was worse, had grown comfortable in it. . . .

The healing I had sought was at hand all the time. I had not accepted it, but it was there. (Kemper, 1977, p. 96)

Negativism and depression have a way of perpetuating themselves unless something intervenes to break the pattern of thought and behavior (Dobson, 1974). The individual needs to be helped to redirect his thought patterns onto the good and positive and redirect mental energies toward social contacts and other appropriate activities.

The individual who is in the succumbing phase needs to be assisted in setting realistic attainable goals. According to Cholden, the successful accomplishment of these goals and activities facilitates the adjusting process.

It is possible to hasten the movement out of the depressed state by the judicious use of activities and tasks. The patient will often get a "lift" after he has successfully accomplished some task he believed difficult at first. Such a task might be simply the ability to navigate correctly to the bathroom, or correctly writing a letter with the help of a script board. However, if he is presented with an overambitious task which he cannot accomplish, the depression may be intensified. An example of such a task is the beginning of teaching braille while the patient is still depressed. (Cholden, 1958, pp. 81-82)

Similarly, appropriate attainable goals and activities can be established for the socially traumatized person. His movement toward withdrawal and depression during this phase can be impeded or reversed when he begins to understand that the source of the stigma is not to be found in himself or his blindness but instead is to be found in the others' faulty and erroneous attitudes toward blindness. Role playing the traumatizing incident to a more satisfactory conclusion, encouraging the individual to explain the source of the stigma to a friend, or restructuring the devaluating and derogatory experience within a more controlled and supportive environment are a few activities that can foster a healthier understanding of a response to social traumas.

The succumbing negativism and depression do not immediately disappear nor are they forever banished. Nevertheless, the breaking of the old thought and behavior pattern with appropriate alternatives does point the individual in the right direction. Schulz (1980) maintained that as the blinded individual "discovers that he can again become a competent and useful person, the depressive mood will gradually lift and he will again resemble the person he was prior to the loss of sight" (p. 39).

> In some ways, learning to mingle with people after one has lost one's sight is rather like playing a game. There is really nothing tragic about it, if you don't let yourself feel that there is. Certain challenges present themselves, and either you give up and refuse to play or you sharpen your wits to win. (Dahl, 1962, p. 141)

Another role of the professional is to help keep the individual's analysis of the "losses" realistic. The unrealistic ones must be challenged and convincingly disproved. The realistic ones must be confronted with their appropriate solutions of adaptive aids or techniques. The medical facts must be clarified to provide the individual with a better understanding of the eye condition and its prognosis.

A word of caution is in order about the use of social comparisons as a therapeutic technique. Negative repercussions are possible in either of two ways. While the professional is trying to compare the individual's situation with someone who appears to be "less fortunate," the individual is just as likely to compare himself with some "more fortunate" and thus intensify his depression. In certain situations, the mere suggestion of the concept of "less fortunate" or "more fortunate" implies a gradation of human value and worth, a most untenable position. However, if the individual himself happens to use the social comparison approach, the professional may simply want to acknowledge that an important step has been taken. Fox used the social comparison approach when he compared himself to a soldier who had been a prisoner of war for three years.

Being next to him made me realize, for the first time, just how lucky I was. It would take that man years to get back to normal, if he ever did. Up until that time I had thought so much about myself, I had not realized that there were many veterans that were much worse off than I. . . . I spent quite a while thinking about that, and was thoroughly ashamed of myself for the self-pity I had allowed to take hold of me at times. I'm glad I had that experience; it did a lot to straighten me out and make me start thinking right. (Fox, 1946, p. 84)

Many have found that group therapy under the direction of a trained counselor can be very effective (Miller, 1971; Routh, 1970; Welsh, 1982). Emerson (1981), after observing a change from self-depreciation and depression to self-acceptance and readjustment among members of her low vision group, asked what accounted for the change in their attitude. Support received from group peers, the opportunity to talk through their problems, and insights gained into some reasons for their own depression were some of the replies given.

It is important to observe that throughout the first four phases of the adjusting process the traumatized person is experiencing emotional turmoil and intellectual confusion. A temporary regression to an egocentric concern about the practical problems being faced is natural and normal. Because of this self-centeredness, he is in no condition to receive or respond to active intervention by the professional. As a result, the role of the professional during the first four phases could best be described as passively supportive. A summary of previously discussed recommendations illustrates the nature of this passive support. They include the suggestions that the professional—

1. provide emotional support and physical comfort;
2. be a good, understanding listener;
3. assist the individual to redirect his mental energies off himself and onto other people and activities;
4. gently confront the individual with the reality of the trauma if he persists with a variety of avoidance behaviors;
5. provide feedback to clarify realistic from unrealistic "losses";

6. assist the individual to set some realistic, attainable goals;
7. provide convincing evidence that a full and satisfying life as a blind person is possible;
8. provide an opportunity for the individual to interact with a blind role model;
9. interpret the dynamics of the adjusting process to family members and friends.

During the succumbing phase, the traumatized individual has reached the emotional low of the entire adjusting process. He is ready to begin the uphill struggle to regain feelings of adequacy and worth, to regain self-acceptance and self-esteem. The first tasks of the turn-around are the reassessment of one's identity, value, and goals and the reaffirmation of the possibilities of life as a visually impaired person.

PHASE FIVE: REASSESSMENT AND REAFFIRMATION

"My turning point," "Life is still worth living"

One day, however, I sensed within myself a small unrest. It was faint, indefinite, vague, as it nudged me. Something was disturbing the dark, the silence. In a bewildered kind of way I sought to identify it. Was this sheer boredom with the constant monotony of everything—was it some belated curiosity about my predicament—was it, perhaps, some tiny seed of decency planted in me years and years before and now stirring to life? I could not say. . . .

Came the inner query: Do you want to be brought back into life, to be revived, resuscitated? Immediately self-pity and inertia replied: let me be. A wiser, calmer voice asked: Is that what you really want? . . . I knew that I did not want to quit. . . .

Most of all I knew I wanted to protect, to nurture the small spark that continued to stir within me. . . . A sense of quietude came over me but it was not the quietude of despair and abandonment which had so lately and so fully possessed me. Indeed, this seemed to be a quietude of waiting. (McCoy, 1963, pp. 27-28)

Regarding the period of reassessment, Giarratana-Oehler (1976) stated that "as the individual is grieving and commencing the process of rehabilitation, he is also beginning a process of re-evaluation" (p. 238). The discouragement, self-pity, and anger of the mourning and succumbing phases begin to recede. The reassessment phase of the adjusting process is the period of time when an individual examines and reconsiders the meaning of life: his basic assumptions, values, beliefs, priorities, and habitual patterns of behavior. During this time, his self-concept undergoes careful scrutiny. He analyzes his personal attributes to determine which need to be replaced, which need to be modified, and which can remain unchanged. Most discover sooner or later that the majority of personal attributes remain untouched or only slightly influenced by the many traumas of blindness. There is, then, a reaffirmation of life and of self.

> I now wanted to seek a new life, no longer concerned with eyes or cures, but a life in the making, built on the remnants of old wrecks and aborted starts, though free of remorse. . . .
> I had now said it all in an ordered sequence: from knowing I'd be blind to experiencing it, from denial to anger to grief, facing it on different levels, joining it, fighting it, pretending it didn't exist or that I could make it all go away. The time for synthesis had arrived, because the sum total of the ignorance and impotence of the various systems I'd explored had finally liberated me from hope. (Potok, 1980, pp. 259, 266)

In the midst of the negativism and apparent hopelessness of the succumbing phase, one searches for solutions, for alternative courses of action. However, the withdrawal, depression, anger, and bitterness of the succumbing phase impede the ability to view objectively all possible alternatives.

> Frustration at every turn, all day, everything just too impossible. . . .
> Affliction—any loss of faculties or what gave life sense—is abominable; admit it; wail, rail, shake your fist—that's what I call healthy.
> Indefinitely? You want to go on raging like that for maybe twenty-some years?
> No.
> Well then. You said a while back you didn't want to get used to it.
> Certainly not. Categorically.
> So you reject the only three alternatives. 1) Get used to it, meaning resigned, maybe just forgetting part of every day how different your expectations once were. 2) Be cheerful, think of the good blah blah

blah as per therapy manual (I guess, have never seen one). 3) Keep raging. Of course there's a fourth, blowing your brains out, but you don't seem to be considering that for some reason. (Clark, 1977, pp. 222-223)

None of the four alternatives are palatable or desirable. As is so often true, Clark was unable to recognize or comprehend a fifth alternative, that of learning to live a full and satisfying life as a person who happens to be blind.

The recognition and comprehension of the fifth alternative is frequently described as "the turning point." The meaning of life becomes one of the first issues to be resolved. This resolution becomes the basis of a new beginning; it provides the impetus and motivation that carries one through the rest of the adjusting process. It requires "a reevaluation of the meaning of life involving a reconsideration of the relative importance of significant values" (Wright, 1960, p. 46). The reevaluation usually results in a reaffirmation of life and its possibilities. After clearing the succumbing and depression debris away, the reaffirmation of life provides a firm foundation for the renovation process.

The future, including future blindness, seemed a challenge to which I was now wholly committed, and this challenge transformed my view of the world. Graduation from Princeton, a meaningless formality toward which I had been stumbling with half a heart, now seemed the very symbol of my first step toward this new world, and I no longer felt the old adolescent fear of failure. In short, I wanted to live as I had never wanted to live before. (Putnam, 1952, pp. 18-19)

Reassessment for the congenitally blind may not manifest itself as dramatically but may emerge as a natural outgrowth of adolescent unrest. The quest for the meaning to life frequently includes the search for an explanation for one's blindness, a search for the answer to the question "Why me?"

State laws now require that silver nitrate must be put in the eyes of all newborn babies. Even now I dare not linger long over the idea that had I been born twenty-five years later, I need not have been blind. When I first realized the full importance of this truth, I was torn by spiritual conflict and bitterness. But I knew I must live at peace with myself. I must live in a world of hope and progress.

> I must search out an explanation for my affliction which would be adequate to my spiritual needs. The thought that the carelessness or ignorance of a doctor had caused my blindness, brought only rebellion. (Brown, 1958, p. 38)

Sometimes there are individuals who are either unable or unwilling to accept the verdicts of reassessment and continue a perpetual search for the meaning of life without ever resolving the questions they continue to ask. The intellectual pursuit of questions that are never resolved is an unhealthy avoidance mechanism. While giving the appearance of an honest search, it may simply be a mask or disguise for lack of emotional self-acceptance.

Identity Crisis

One of the next issues to be resolved is the question of one's identity. This is not unlike the adolescent's search for his identity, "Who am I?" The many traumas of blindness precipitate doubts about one's identity.

First, both the congenitally and recently blind struggle from time to time with incorporating the attribute of blindness into their self-concept.

> I hoped against hope that the blindness would go away. My high school junior year was the most difficult of my life. All the defenses I had built up around myself fell away and I finally came to the full realization that I was going to be different for the rest of my life. My blindness was real. It wasn't going to go away. (Sperber, 1976, p. 74)

The acceptance of the fact of blindness as one of the personal attributes in the self-concept must occur before any possibility of further adequate adjustment can take place. Cholden suggested that the blind person "must learn to accept his blindness as a condition of his life, as he accepts the relative weakness of his left hand and the air that he breathes. Otherwise, he will be unable to wholeheartedly enter into the re-educational activities that can restore him to a satisfying and productive life" (p. 18).

One measure of acceptance is the extent to which the individual identifies with the blind (Klich and Wierig, 1971) rather than the sighted with respect to visual behaviors and activity. Good adjustment reflects identification with the sighted in all ways other than blindness-related attributes. If the individual attempts to function "as if" he could see, if he gives the pretense of being able to see, he will continue to experience uncomfortable discrepancies in his life. Furthermore, "denial can take a passive form in which the patient verbalizes his acceptance of his condition but does nothing to adjust to it" (Dover, 1959, p. 336).

In the second place, the resolution of the identity crisis includes a reaffirmation of the self. He comes to recognize himself as essentially the same person as before the trauma with a majority of his personal attributes intact, untouched by the trauma. The degree to which blindness remains the focal point of attention is the degree to which the individual will continue to feel essentially different.

> My inmost dislike has always been for seeming different from the rest of my fellow men. Every act of my life has been in the direction of making myself as close to the norm as possible. I therefore could not now accept the notion that I had suddenly become inherently peculiar, and that is the feeling which drove me forward to reattaining as much of my old position as I could. (Chevigny, 1946, p. 258)

Reassessing Assets, Goals, and Values

The reassessment phase also involves the process of determining realistically one's strengths and limitations. The analysis requires that the individual be able to differentiate among three types of limitations: (1) the perceived limitations that are unrealistic, resulting from "spread," (2) the temporary limitations that can be circumvented by learning the proper use of adaptive aids and techniques, and (3) the more permanent limitations that must be accepted as unalterable. The recently traumatized is frequently unable to make this differentiation without assistance. Yet, any movement toward more positive appraisals is a step in the right direction.

> Until my arrival at Morristown, I had been trying to walk backward into the future, with my mind closed to everything but the magnitude

of my loss. Now I was starting to think in terms of my blessings. Perhaps I was beginning to grow up. (Clifton, 1963, p. 70)

"The insecurity of the person who tries to forget and conceal his disability is yet further increased because he does not allow himself to clarify what he can and cannot do.... The person does not allow himself to clarify his behavior possibilities because, in order to do so, he must first be able to acknowledge, 'this is my limitation'" (Wright, 1960, pp. 48-49). Recognition of one's assets and limitations is a prerequisite to adequate adjusting behavior.

> Only then will he realistically be able to study the requirements of different situations toward his more able functioning in them. Only then will demarcation between what he can and cannot do become more sharply defined. Only then will he realize that confidence in the self which is essential to the adequate meeting of new situations that inevitably present themselves. (Wright, 1960, p. 49)

> With this understanding of God's promise to strengthen me I prayed for the courage to hold firmly to my resolution, made so long ago, never to become a burden to those around me. Next I began to catalogue my personal assets; if I were to succeed in climbing the wall that stood before me I would need every asset I could muster. (Carver, 1961, p. 157)

The reassessment phase also involves a reconsideration of goals and values. The process of analyzing and modifying one's goals and values does not terminate with "acceptance of the fact of blindness" but continues throughout life. Some goals are blocked, others can be substituted for the blocked goals. Some goals are not blocked and can be reached directly. Still others can be reached by circumventing the barrier (Cohn, 1961). The values that guide the selection of one's goals and the means to those goals undergo scrutiny and possible revision. High priority values that are incompatible with blindness must be lowered in priority, modified, or replaced (see Chapter 5).

> You may say it's impossible for a nine-year-old to be grown-up, but that night I became an adult. It's amazing what can happen to you when you're faced with something like a lifetime of blindness.
> ... That night I lay there and argued the pros and cons of a life of

dependence on others or a life of independence. Of course, the argument was handled at a nine-year-old level, but the problem was wrestled with nonetheless. . . .

It was very, very late when I finally determined that I wanted to be independent. . . .

I have never really been even tempted to change my mind since that night so long ago. I grew up that night and made a choice. I would not be a blind man in a blind world. (Krents, 1972, pp. 93-94)

With the analysis of one's assets and liabilities, the newly restructured goals and values must be put to the test of everyday living. Capitalizing on one's assets, a person can begin immediately to set and achieve some realistic attainable goals as a way of arresting the succumbing negativism.

Through this reality testing, formerly perceived "losses" may no longer be considered losses at all. Fox, who had thought himself incapable of being a good father, discovered through an experience of horseback riding with his six-year-old son that the reality was quite different.

Being with that boy did more than any treatment I received to restore my confidence. Any dad dreams of being able to teach his son how to hunt and fish; of going camping with him, and teaching him the rudiments of good sportsmanship. With my son's help, I learned I could do all these things, even without vision. . . . In other words, the close feeling that should exist between father and son will not be denied me because of my blindness. If I use my head and a little ingenuity, we can be as close as any other boy and his dad. (Fox, 1946, p. 152)

The immediate attainment of some short-term goals and the successful accomplishment of some daily activities can have a positive impact on one's self-esteem, self-confidence, and general outlook on the future. The turning point from depression for Fitzgerald's (1970) blind subjects "was associated with increased self-esteem from attempting and mastering self-sufficient acts, and with the establishment of important interpersonal relationships with caregivers and other blind persons" (p. 373).

Role of Hope and Faith

"Hope is a feeling that may accompany any stage but

shock. It is the one underlying factor that can motivate a client to recognize and accept the change" (VanderKolk, 1981, p. 143). Hope can motivate a person to work toward bettering his situation if he really believes that things can improve (Schulz, 1980). Like the analysis of assets, goals, and values, hope must also be based in reality. While realistic hope can motivate toward better adjusting, unrealistic hope for miraculous cures and scientific inventions inhibits the adjusting process.

> After a minute of, I hope, silent despair, I realized I wasn't going to get anywhere by lying there filled with self-pity. What I had to do was to plan my life to overcome my handicap.... I did begin to realize that there was no reason I should not be able to live a full and happy life. (Fox, 1946, pp. 28-29)

Although the poem to which Blackhall refers has not been reprinted here, the following excerpt expresses his honesty regarding a conviction of hope and joy even in the midst of a deep hurt. Furthermore, he maintains that hope and joy can be found in every human trauma.

> I ask you to believe that I have written this poem in that spirit of honesty. In it, because it is sincere, there is something of the doubt and insecurity and something of the deep hurt which one cannot entirely escape or disguise in a situation like mine. But more important than this, if my poem is successful in saying what I want it to say, there is something of the hope and joy which all of us find in every human crisis. It is always there and it is ours for the asking. (Blackhall, 1962, p. 127)

One's faith or one's relationship to God can have a positive influence, in that it can sustain a person through a crisis. However, sustaining faith is not generated out of trauma. To be effective, sustaining faith must already be in existence and active before the crisis.

> Without my faith in God, I doubt that I should have been able to travel that road myself with any degree of success. It is a faith that has been my sure guide for many years, one which I am glad to say was acquired before blindness assailed me. (Bretz, 1940, p. 192)

> I know that God could have taken my life as easily as He took my sight. During my first moments of depression I wondered why He had not done so; then it came to me that He must have some reason. What

that reason is, I don't know; but I am sure, as I go on through life, it will be revealed to me.

The only thing left for me is to abide by His decision. I can be a man and accept things the way they are, or I can pity myself to the extent of blaming Him for an unjust decision. I believe praying for the return of my vision would be simply asking Him to change His mind, and who am I to question His decision, by asking Him to change His mind? (Fox, 1946, pp. 115-116)

Role of the Professional

The support network of family and professionals continues to play an important role during the reassessment and reaffirmation phase. The person who has just experienced the negativism of succumbing and depression needs strong evidence for the reaffirmation of life and self. A great deal of convincing proof is required before a drastic remodeling of the self-concept can take place in a positive direction (Rogers, 1951). It is the rare individual who can attain the convincing evidence alone; he needs the support network (see Chapter 9).

The change we have to make is like learning to drive a car up a long hill. If there is someone with us who can show how to shift gears, taking the hill is easy. I confess that, traveling alone, I stalled the engine a number of times, but the car never turned over, nor did it slide downhill. (Bretz, 1940, p. 143)

The professional has a responsibility to help foster a positive frame of mind. "The quality of life need not be compromised because of a visual defect. The most important element in a child's eventual appreciation of his existence is the harmony of thought and action that results from promoting strengths rather than deficits" (Mangold, 1982, p. 94). Encouraging a positive outlook can be accomplshed by appropriate example and discussion as well as by providing appropriate literature. The resolution to refrain from self-pity and to avoid playing "if only" games is illustrated by Blackhall.

I look back now and think how fortunate I am that I have been able to shut out from my mind, to abandon it as soon as it was born, every thought which began with, "If only," or "I wish." Once we give credence to the thought that life has dealt a little harshly with us, we are not far from believing that we deserve something better. From that point onwards, if we don't watch out, we begin to feel sorry for ourselves. And nothing worthwhile, in all the history of mankind, ever came from self-pity. . . .

What is the use of my saying, "If only it had been different"? It's not different; it's like this! (Blackhall, 1962, pp. 124-126)

With respect to the reality of blindness and its implications, the professional dare not hedge or equivocate. The visually impaired person's reaction to being identified as "blind" is an indicator of the degree to which he has incorporated the attribute of blindness into his self-concept. Frank, factual information about the person's condition and prognosis has to be confronted and accepted before any further adjusting can occur. There are degrees of acceptance, and a sensitive professional should be alert to the indicators of the person's degree of acceptance and of his readiness for even greater acceptance.

Certainly, in my teens when for the first time I became aware of something of the true significance of being blind, I urgently wanted to know the answers to two questions: was there any hope of a cure in my lifetime, and was there anything hereditary about the complaint. These were overriding considerations for a time. Then in a few seconds I got a firm "no" to both from an eye specialist who had known my case from the time I was a few months old.

Since then I have not been very much concerned with the physical fact of blindness. I have had no choice but to devote most of my attentions to the more practical matter of learning to bypass the everyday difficulties which are inseparable from lack of sight, and recognizing those times when I must be prepared to accept help from other people. (Edwards, 1962, pp. 7-8)

To help the individual assess his own strengths and limitations, the professional must provide realistic feedback without any hint of patronizing or condescension. If the professional and family members treat him as a person with equal dignity and worth, then he is more likely to view himself in a similar manner. The best feedback comes from placing the blind person in as normal a situation as possible so that he can confront the realities of life, thus facilitating a more accurate assessment of strengths and limitations.

Sheltered or overprotective treatment results in distorted or inflated estimates of one's personal attributes. When the blind person is still emerging from the negative, succumbing phase, the tendency is to focus on the perceived limitations in order to clarify them. Thereafter, the trend should be to focus more and more on the assets or strengths.

> As I sat, I made up my mind about one thing. I was doing the best I could, and I wouldn't let myself dwell on any imperfections. This would only bring on frustration and make the work much less satisfactory. I would accept my limitations, but first I would make absolutely sure what my limitations were. (Dahl, 1962, p. 113)

Hamachek (1971) described four constructive compensatory behaviors beneficial to the person with perceived inferior status or perceived limitations.
1. Select satisfying and useful endeavors that reflect a person's strengths.
2. Stimulate and channel the individual's ambitions into concrete efforts permitting him to work hard at what he can do rather than allowing him to fret about what he cannot do.
3. Encourage the attractiveness of the personality to show by developing good interpersonal skills.
4. Appreciate one's relative advantages by emphasizing the positive rather than the negative (p. 239).

Other guidelines the professional will find useful are presented by Wright (1960). The following processes help to foster a positive change in one's value priorities, which enable the individual to overcome "the feeling of shame and inferiority resulting from disability as a value loss" (p. 108).

1. Enlarge the scope of values:

> Enlarging the scope of values means the emotional realization of the existence of other values. . . . We do know that the values presumed lost may be perceived in a new way, in which their essential aspects are retained and not in fact denied. . . . The person becomes aware of his own assets or abilities, and particularly that these enable him to participate in his own way, as others can in their own way, in the multivaried world. (pp. 108-114)

2. Subordinate physique: Subordinating physique can happen in one of two ways.

> In the first of these, physical appearance matters less and in the second, physical ability matters less. . . . This shift is facilitated when the person is convinced of the fundamental importance of nonphysique values, such as kindness, wisdom, effort, cooperativeness. . . . Physical appearance and ability were both subordinated to personality factors within the person over which he has more control. (pp. 116-117)

3. Contain the disability effects:

> Not all of life is influenced, let alone determined by disability. The person with a disability must be encouraged to pinpoint the values now lost to him so that they become but dots in the large map of the world, in which vast areas remain relatively intact and accessible. He will then realize that he is not a disabled person but a person with a disability, that life has a multitude of meanings, opportunities, and frustrations, only some of which are disability-connected. (p. 128)

4. Transform comparative values into asset values:

> If the evaluation is based on comparison with a standard, the person is said to be invoking comparative values. . . . On the other hand, if the evaluation arises from the qualities inherent in the object of judgment itself, the person is said to be invoking asset values. What matters is the object of judgment in a setting that has its own intrinsic purposes and demands. The person's reaction is then based upon how appropriately the situational demands are fulfilled rather than on comparison with a predetermined standard. (p. 129)

The need to share with another is present whether verbalized or not. The role of the professional involves assisting the socially or physically traumatized person to think out and work through the reassessment and reaffirmation phase. Most often, the itinerant teacher in school or the rehabilitation teacher in the home will work through these issues gradually on an individual basis. Much of this work can also be accomplished in a discussion group or mutual support group (Emerson, 1981; Galler, 1981; Welsh, 1982). Members of Emerson's low vision group were encouraged to express and analyze their concerns, clarify their value priorities, discover realistic solutions, and develop a concern for other members in the group. She reported that most group members moved from shock and depression, through other adjusting phases and finally to readjustment, which was marked by self-confrontation, redefinition, and acceptance of a modified identity and revised self-concept. Kemper recognized his need for such a group.

> I am not alone, I am in a large group. But the group of us waiting in the lobby did not know we were a group. Each one of us was fighting his or her own battle, privately. We should have compared notes, not troubled glances. (Kemper, 1977, p. 28)

The role of the professional, according to Routh (1970) is to assist the visually impaired person to cope with his social and physical environment and, where necessary, to restructure it; to establish realistic, attainable goals; to gain insights into himself and his blindness; to clarify his attitudes, feelings, and emotional reactions to his problems; and to determine the motivational factors that contribute to the adjusting process. Routh maintained that the main purpose of a rehabilitation program "is to have the blind client make a more positive, realistic appraisal of himself, his handicap, his emotional assets and liabilities, by working through some of those factors connected with his feelings and attitudes" (p. 19).

The period of reassessment and reaffirmation in the adjusting process is described as a turning point toward a more positive outlook. During this phase, the visually impaired person reconsiders the meaning of life, engages in a reaffirmation of life and of self, searches for an explanation of the trauma, negotiates a resolution of the identity crisis, and clarifies his assets, goals, and values. Some of these tasks are actually begun during the previous succumbing phase and some are not fully achieved until the individual is well into the next phase of coping and mobilization.

PHASE SIX: COPING AND MOBILIZATION

"I can," "Some things I do in a different way"

Having initiated the process toward acceptance of the unpleasant reality and the reassessment of one's assets, goals, and values, the individual is now prepared for the coping and mobilization phase. Coping refers to the process of learning to manage the demands of one's physical and social environment. It involves the acquisition of new skills and the mobilization of internal and external resources (Dover, 1959). "'Adjustment' suggests accommodation to pressures, while 'coping' implies active mastery" (Lazarus, 1969, p. 209). Coping is the adjustable aspect of the trauma, a time when the individual directs his "physic energy to the solution of real problems of living " (Blank, 1957, p. 14). Coping leads to habilitation or rehabilitation and is a prerequisite to self-acceptance (Wright, 1960).

The characteristics of successful coping that create a climate for self-acceptance and self-esteem include the following:

1. Emphasis on what a person *can do.*
2. Areas of life in which the person can participate are seen as worthwhile.
3. The person is perceived as playing an *active role* in molding his life constructively.
4. The accomplishments of the person are appreciated in terms of their benefits to the person and others and not primarily depreciated because they fall short of some irrelevant standard.
5. The negative aspects of the person's life, such as the pain that is suffered or difficulties that exist, are felt to be manageable.
6. Managing difficulties, in one sense, means overcoming them or ameliorating them through the application of medical procedures, the use of prostheses and other aids, learning new skills, and environmental accommodations (social, legal, economic, etc.).
7. Managing difficulties also means *living on satisfactory terms* with one's limitations (although the disability may be regarded as a nuisance and sometimes a burden). Above all this means viewing the disability as nondevaluating and seeking satisfaction in terms of one's assets. (Wright, 1974, p. 115)

Coping Strategies

Coping requires "making an assessment of a) residual

capacities of the body and b) the goals and values of the person" and bringing "these two sets of factors into satisfying relationship with one another" (Jourard, 1963, p. 414). To illustrate, Boswell found that there was little satisfaction in developing adaptive skills without meaningful goals.

> The problem was my own lack of ability to get with the business of being blind. I didn't feel that I was accomplishing a thing, but that hardly surprised me because I had no real goals that I was the least bit interested in achieving. (Boswell, 1969, p. 110)

Lambert, West, and Carlin (1981) suggested that coping or adjusting with blindness involved "thinking out" and "acting on" an appropriate context or life situation in two ways: (1) "make substitutions for major elements of an existing context" such as a new home location or a new career, and (2) "rearrange or redefine relationships among elements of an existing context" such as another way to travel (p. 194).

Substitution is a timeless coping strategy; it has been used throughout all history. The rejected suitor finds another. The person who cannot play tennis because of blindness seeks another recreation outlet: skiing, jogging, or bike riding. One can appreciate the replacement for its own value without depreciating or devaluating the replaced (Schulz, 1980).

Another ageless coping strategy involves attacking the source of the problem. If a blind person feels inadequate or devaluated because he is unable to perform certain functions, then he can learn to use new tools and techniques, thus restoring his sense of competence. Since old familiar ways of doing things frequently have become habitual, it requires time and effort to replace these old habits with new ones.

> An orderly brought me some shaving soap and an old three-piece Gillette razor. I ran him out, closed the door, and started the operation. Soon after I began, I laughed. I was standing at the washbasin just as I always had, and I was looking into the mirror. If anyone had been watching me, they might not have realized that I really didn't need that mirror. I didn't need to rely on Pete or anyone else to shave me, either. (Boswell, 1969, p. 76)

> In this early period of readjustment I was amazed and strange as it may sound, intensely interested in learning to perform silly little everyday actions in a new way. Nor was it just learning something new. Quite the contrary, it was learning to do the old thing in a new way, and simultaneously learning to forget the former method. (Bretz, 1940, p. 44)

Increased proficiency in these coping skills tends to foster a sense of accomplishment and pride, to enhance one's self-esteem.

> One day after I had learned the fundamentals of the Braille system and had practiced enough so that I could actually read, I was informed that we had copies of the *Readers' Digest* in our library. While thumbing through one issue, I came across an article entitled "Three Cheers for George Washington High." My interest was suddenly aroused. My high school had received national recognition in an article in the *Readers' Digest* earlier that year. I had asked several people to find a copy of the magazine and read the article to me at the time it was first published, but I was never successful. . . .
>
> Though my Braille reading speed was slow, I could now read the whole article by myself. I started the article during my regular Braille lesson that afternoon and took the book with me to read on my own. . . .
>
> "I made it!" I almost whispered victoriously. "I read the whole thing." . . . It was a thrilling and memorable experience. (Cordellos, 1981, p. 48)

On the other hand, if a blind person feels inadequate or devaluated because of society's derogatory attitudes about blindness, then he must attack the source of that problem. The prevailing negative attitudes that may result in injustice, discrimination, and prejudice can be assaulted by educational campaigns through mass media, by legislative provisions that seek to protect the rights of the handicapped, and by aggressive and even militant protest movements. None, however, is as effective in changing an individual's attitude as the slow and tedious process of getting to know and appreciate each person one by one. (See Chapter 4 on types of relationships.)

Another effective coping strategy is to concentrate more on positive aspects of an apparent liability, making it work to one's advantage. While most would agree that blindness is not advantageous, there are some situations in which it can be turned to one's benefit. The maladaptive counterpart of this coping strategy, that of inappropriately using blindness, is discussed later in this section, along with other maladaptive coping strategies.

> Suddenly, . . . came the idea that blindness, a handicap in many fields of medicine as it was in day camp, could be an advantage in psychiatry. I felt I could bring a special empathy to patients coping with such stresses as phobias and difficulties in interpersonal relationships as well as to emotional problems of the disabled. My handicap would be a strength. Instead of competing with sighted people on their ground, I could create a ground of my own where *they* would have to work twice as hard to keep up with *my* understanding.
>
> The road to validating that idea has been winding and rocky and long. Along the way I have developed a companion to my precept that everybody is handicapped. The companion idea is that the people most likely to succeed are those who have a knack for turning their handicaps into advantages. (Hartman and Asbell, 1978, p. 92)

The mobilization aspect of this phase involves the acknowledgement of the need for, the search for, the recognition of, and the effective utilization of personal, interpersonal, and institutional resources. Personal resources are one's own strengths and assets; interpersonal resources refer to the support network of family, friends, and professionals; and institutional resources include schools, agencies, and/or organizations of and for the blind. Mobilization is the "active use of personal and outside resources for enriching one's functioning at every level" (Dover, 1959, p. 336). The vast array of knowledge about one's resources and the ability to orchestrate them effectively for maximum benefit takes a great deal of time and effort to acquire and develop them to the fullest.

Adaptive Coping Behaviors and Attitudes

The process of helping a person to learn to cope with the physical and social traumas of blindness requires a diverse approach. There are times when concentrated individual instruction is best and other times when the interactive group instruction is preferable. There are advantages to each of the work settings: the home with its more natural setting and potential for family involvement; the school with its immediate access to any possible personal, peer, or staff difficulties and their potential solutions; and the rehabilitation center with its specialized facilities and equipment, trained staff, and opportunity for group interaction. Programs that foster maximum adaptive coping behaviors must be comprehensive and thoroughly planned (Cholden, 1958; Jones, 1980; Moos and Tsu, 1977; Parad and Caplan, 1965; Routh, 1970). To be effective, they must address the three areas of physical, cognitive, and affective.

1. Physical: to enable the VI—
   a. to obtain the best possible medical attention;
   b. to secure the best possible low vision examination and, when indicated, to secure proper low vision aids and training.
2. Cognitive: to enable the VI—
   a. to gain an accurate understanding of the problem and to secure all relevant information, e.g. nature of disease, explanation of attitudes, legislative provisions;
   b. to acquire and to use adaptive aids and techniques properly;
   c. to secure and manage personal, interpersonal, and institutional resources;
   d. to develop good interpersonal skills particularly as they relate to assistance offered by others or sought and received by self (see Chapter 9);
   e. to prepare for any possible future traumas by rehearsing potential alternative outcomes;
   f. to continue analyzing and revising goals and values in keeping with newfound abilities and interests.
3. Affective: to enable the VI—
   a. to put the "seriousness" of the trauma into proper perspective;
   b. to manage one's feelings and emotions;
   c. to develop healthy attitudes toward blindness and toward the demands of the physical and social envi-

ronment including a positive attitude toward "the sighted";

d. to develop a wholesome, positive attitude toward self, capitalizing on one's assets and living contentedly within one's real limitations for a full and satisfying life.

The reward of social approval for meeting others' expectations is a powerful motivating force. If the expected role is that of a helpless, dependent blind person, then there is social approval in playing that role. If, however, the expected role is that of a competent, assertive, self-directed person, who is visually impaired, then meeting those expectations is rewarding. Gergan (1971) maintained that "rewards and punishments associated with a concept affect the evaluative connotation of the concept. Thus, if a person is rewarded for behaving in a particular role, he should come to prefer it and should receive gratification for thinking of himself in terms of the role" (p. 57).

For some, self-expectations are as powerful a motivator as the expectations of others, if not even more powerful. If self-expectations include competence and independence, then the mastering of normal daily activities contributes to improved self-respect and self-acceptance.

> He is learning that he can improve his situation and that in coping with the many "little things" he is coping with the biggest thing of all: gaining self-respect. It has been said that working with daily-activity skills is the basis for all subsequent rehabilitation processes. This is as true for the restoration of self-respect as it is for the restoration of physical independence. (Wright, 1960, p. 65)

Successes in daily tasks and relationships are equally important for children. "Confrontation with reality in an atmosphere of warmth and acceptance is imperative if one is to get an accurate view of self. False praise for poor performance is seen by the student as a sham. Here, it is emphasized that students must be provided real experiences in which they can have success and from which they can draw the inference that they are successful" (LaBenne and Greene, 1969, p. 32).

Coping requires effort and effort requires energy. Effort alone without knowing how or what do to simply consumes energy without being productive. "While effective coping with stress always uses energy, the amount required can be reduced in direct proportion to the number and degree of relevant skills that can be applied to the coping effort" (Stringer, 1971, pp. 16-17).

Frequently the recently blind who are still in the process of learning new coping skills complain that "everything" now takes more time and effort, more physical, mental, and emotional energy.

> Sometimes the things that seem most difficult to you are the ones you did not expect would give you any trouble. You have to learn to be patient and persistent, for everything you do will need the expenditure of far more energy and effort than the ordinary person finds necessary. (Pierce, 1944, p. 125)

However, as the new coping skills are mastered, their performance becomes more routine and normal, requiring less time, effort, and energy than originally thought (Roberts, 1973). In the same respect, the young blind learner requires additional time, energy, and effort before his adaptive skills become normalized, habitualized, and routinized. The more of the coping behaviors that are mastered and utilized, the less effort and energy required to maintain oneself.

> When finality is accepted, one begins to cope with the resulting disorders. When one copes long enough, a new order beings. With the passage of time the new order becomes normalcy. (Kemper, 1977, p. 102)

During the coping phase, the individual will still occasionally revert back to some of his old feelings of self-pity, doubt, and discouragement, but for shorter, less intense, and less frequent periods. This is particularly true each time he encounters an unfamiliar situation or unresolved discrepancy. As his coping behaviors become better established, he should experience less frustration and anxiety regarding his ability to manage himself within his environment. "It has been shown that individuals do not remain in a state of frustration with objects or with facts indefinitely.

Where frustration continues, the inciting sources are people who can be constantly changing and providing new means of frustration" (Riffinburgh, 1967, p. 128).

People in the coping phase of adjusting frequently comment that they feel self-conscious. This is perfectly natural, for they are still experimenting with newly acquired skills in a social setting where it is impossible to determine whether they are being observed. With time and practice, the new becomes normal and natural. When a person is self-conscious, he tends to avoid doing anything that will draw further attention to himself, preferring instead the "safety" of isolation or withdrawal. Of course, isolation precludes all opportunity for requisite practice of the new skills so essential for normalizing one's behavior.

A little confidence gained from a successful experience has a way of generating even more confidence. Increasing confidence and self-esteem in one area can motivate a person to acquire skills in other areas and thus little by little self-esteem grows.

> Golf quickly brought me back into top physical condition, but that was only one of the ways in which it sharpened my life. I took fresh interest in the Braille and typing courses Valley Forge offered, and my confidence shot sky-high. There was some hope for me to make a strong comeback, after all—thanks to golf, and what being good at it meant to me. (Boswell, 1969, p. 115)

Maladaptive Coping Behaviors and Attitudes

The tendency to employ maladaptive adjusting behaviors and attitudes may continue to appear during the coping and mobilization phase. Even while a person is learning new coping behaviors, he may employ some of the defense mechanisms to one degree or another. Attempts to manipulate others by trading on his blindness, although natural for a child, become maladaptive if allowed to go unchecked.

> There was, unfortunately, a pie covered with cellophane on the counter. Before I could steer his hands in a different direction, Davey's fingers had encountered the smooth crisp paper and he was eager to see what was inside. I pulled his hands away, explaining that it was a pie and he must not touch it. . . .

"I wanted to see that pie," Davey insisted again as we went out the door, "I wanted to."

"Now listen," I said, and I kept my voice firm, but I tried to be reasonable too. "You might as well learn right now, Davey, that there are some things in this world that you cannot touch, and that pie was one of them. We simply can't let you handle things that other people want to eat. It isn't sanitary, and you just can't."

His lip stuck out further than ever, and he jerked his hand in disgust.

"That's a fine thing," he said, and his tone was very accusing. "That's a fine thing to say to a little blind boy."

For a minute I was shocked, and then I wanted to laugh. But I didn't dare. Well, it was bound to come, I knew—this trading on his blindness. But I hadn't thought it would come so quickly. (Henderson, 1954, pp. 221-222)

The maladaptive behaviors and attitudes listed below are some of the more commoly mentioned in the literature (Cohn, 1961; Fitzgerald, 1970; Hamachek, 1971; Jourard, 1963; Lambert et al., 1981; Riffenburgh, 1967; Schulz, 1980). Almost everyone, blind or sighted, has, at one time or the other, used one or more of these inappropriate adjusting patterns. There is no need for alarm when they are employed infrequently and superficially; however, intense and habitual use of one or more of them is an indicator of a more severe maladaptive state of adjustment.

1. Maladaptive forms of denial include—
   a. concealing blindness in public, while admitting to oneself the need for coping behavior;
   b. viewing the condition as only temporary, thus minimizing the need for coping skills;
   c. persistent and inappropriate searching for cures, minimizing the need for coping skills;
   d. denying that any barriers exist, maintaining that all goals are attainable.
2. The more passive maladaptive behaviors include—
   a. quitting or giving up, resigning oneself to extreme dependency;
   b. relinquishing decision making, permitting a significant other or an organization to set all goals, values, and standards of behavior;
   c. digging in for a lifetime devoid of satisfactions, a

helpless, empty, and meaningless existence;

d. persisting in willful ignorance about blindness and related coping skills, choosing not to put forth the necessary time and effort.

3. The more assertive maladaptive behaviors include—

a. refusing all assistance, training, aids, or special techniques, preferring the extreme independence of "doing it myself";

b. overcompensating with a desire to prove equality in every situation, the amazing "superblind";

c. reacting with decided superiority and arrogance, needing to prove "I am always right."

4. Other maladaptive behaviors include—

a. understanding what should be done, but either unable or unwilling to follow through or achieve satisfactory coping behaviors;

b. setting goals beyond reasonable possibility of attainment, thus able to blame blindness for one's failure;

c. fantasying or engaging in excessive daydreaming, continuing to play "if only . . ." games;

d. continuing to long for sight;

e. using blindness inappropriately, playing upon the emotions of others for special treatment or favors;

f. attempting to convince others that one is well-adjusted, while projecting his own negative feelings onto others.

Some of the maladaptive coping behaviors can be observed in the following excerpts.

> Night after night, following the endless days at the stand, I'd walk home, eat whatever my mother put out for me, or open a can of beans and eat them cold, then sit in my room. . . .
> What would I think about? Was I sad? Or just disgusted? Or did I pity myself? No, I wasn't sad, exactly, nor did I pity myself. I was plain mad. I took my fate stoically, with a constant, seething determination not to accept it without fighting against it, and the resolution to some day lead a normal life that would allow me to forget my handicap. (Sheppard, 1956, pp. 78-79)

> More and more friends came to our house and no reference was ever made to my blindness. We all acted as though there were nothing

the matter with me. (Bretz, 1940, p. 61)

What she had not learned was how to get on with her blindness. She felt that people around her were embarrassed by her blindness and as a result she was embarrassed. When she would get on a bus, she would put the cane away and refuse to use it on the way home from the bus stop when she got off. Her refusal to accept blindness and her resistance to the cane placed her in such danger that eventually she was forced into acceptance, not because of her own safety but because of the way others who were concerned about her were affected. (Sperber, 1976, p. 107)

Role of the Professional

The role of the professional during the coping and mobilization phase is to facilitate the acquisition of appropriate adjusting behaviors and attitudes. First, accurate information about blindness and its implications must be made available for the required cognitive growth. This information might include facts regarding the medical diagnosis and prognosis of the eye condition, organizations and resources of and for the blind, recreational and vocational possibilities, etc. The second ingredient to facilitate the adjusting process is the development of a sequential program to teach the adaptive skills required for maximum independent functioning. The third ingredient is the affective component, to foster the development of healthy attitudes and feelings toward blindness, self, and others. "Negative or devaluating aspects of disability must be brought to the young person's awareness, along with the coping aspects, by those who know and love him" (Wright, 1960, p. 158).

An appropriate balance among the three ingredients can and should be maintained throughout all activities and discussions. As a general rule, one does not plan a separate lesson for each of the three ingredients but rather addresses all three areas in every lesson. The healthy attitudes and positive feelings that are learned are a by-product of working together on the knowledge and skills. The attitudes and feelings of the professional are observed and assimilated by the blind person, and this occurs usually at the unconscious level. For this reason, it is important that the professional have worked through his own feelings and attitudes toward blindness to a positive resolution so that his verbal and nonverbal projections reveal healthy attitudes and feelings worth modeling.

In recent years a movement known as "consumerism" has gained prominence. As the name implies, the consumers of the service take a more active role in their education and rehabilitation programming. These visually impaired children and adults are active participants in the process of setting their own goals and outlining the strategies for their attainment. In certain situations consumers may be able, through peer counseling, to exert a greater influence than the professional in the lives of fellow consumers, particularly in the affective domain. As a result, the professional will want to take advantage of opportunities to provide occasions for consumers to interact with each other.

The most concentrated growth opportunities are provided by schools or orientation/rehabilitation centers for the blind. In addition to the trained staff and specialized facility, the day-long program of classes and activities provides ample opportunity for interaction at both the formal and informal levels. Bauman (1954b) was able to demonstrate that rehabilitation training accomplished more than growth simply in knowledge and skills. After a twelve-week training program, the clients demonstrated significant improvement in their feelings of adequacy, attitudes regarding blindness, social competency, and emotional stability.

Unfortunately, itinerant teachers employed in the public schools and rehabilitation teachers working in the home have more difficulty structuring group interaction among their students or clients. It would be advisable to set up lessons specifically for small group instruction. The instructional topics can vary from planning and preparing a meal to legal rights of the handicapped. Yank (1968) reported that the success of the small instructional group of adults was due to an "atmosphere of gentle competition; sharing of knowledge and problems; formation of a close knit group with a unity of purpose" (p. 316). Group membership enhances mutual support and encouragement, accountability to one another and freedom of expression through respect and confidentiality.

Community group activities can also provide the climate for affective growth (Welsh, 1982). This is not to be confused with the therapy groups led by a trained counselor discussed in the "Role of the Professional" of the Succumbing and Depression Phase. Rather, they are professionally-led discussion groups that center on particular topics of interest: hobbies, dining, independence, service to others, relationships, etc. The focus of these groups should be on the understanding and management of problems related to blindness, superficial, surface problems, rather than the more deep-seated emotional problems (Routh, 1970). Frequently, the more heterogeneous the group is (the more it represents a wide range of age, amount of vision from fully sighted to totally blind, and recency of visual loss), the more effective is the group. This type of activity permits the professional to interact with the group on a more informal level and also permits interaction among group members. Although growth in social, recreational, and other daily living skills takes place, the growth possibilities in the affective domain are just as important.

Harshbarger (1980), who led a discussion group of elderly visually impaired persons, found that as a result of the group interaction, their depression was alleviated and their self-image, self-acceptance, self-esteem, and self-confidence were improved. The group members learned that their thoughts and feelings, especially about visual impairment, were shared by others in the group, learned to understand other visually impaired persons with a variety of visual losses, and learned to ask their friends and family members for necessary help.

The availability of suitable "models" for sighted children and adults is often taken for granted. However, because of the low incidence of blindness and because blindness limits observation, more time and effort are required to enable blind persons to observe and model appropriate behaviors. There are two types of models to be considered. First, congenitally blind children need appropriate models among their sighted peers to learn the standards of behavior irrespective of sight. Second, both the congenital and adventitious blind need to observe other blind persons who can model healthy coping behaviors and attitudes. It may require a great deal of structuring or manipulating to bring the student or client into contact with an appropriate model who is visually impaired, but the potential results are well worth the effort.

> A man may worry about being blind when he first comes there, but he soon gets over it. When he sees from thirty to fifty men who don't give a darn about their blindness, men who can talk with confidence about the future, men who go out every night of liberty—and any other night they can without being caught—men who can still discuss the Navy's favorite topic—girls—and do it without a trace of self-consciousness because of their blindness, he soon learns that he feels better when he doesn't worry himself about not being able to see. (Fox, 1946, p. 124)

In addition to the blind models available in the community, one can reinforce appropriate adjusting behaviors and attitudes through the judicious use of biographies and autobiographies of visually impaired persons (see References). However, their premature use during any of the previous phases such as mourning or succumbing is likely to be ineffective.

Another vehicle for fostering cognitive growth is that of role playing. Through role playing, one can anticipate some potential social traumas and prepare oneself to meet them by rehearsing in advance. Suggested topics of the role-playing situation are available in other parts of this book: common attitudes about blindness in Chapter 3, types of relationships in Chapter 4, characteristics of high and low self-esteem persons in Chapter 6, and different ways that assistance is offered and received in Chapter 9. Sometimes the professional can take the role of the sighted, while the child or client takes the role of the blind person. At other times, they can reverse their roles. In any case, to be effective, both parties in the role-playing situations must actively involve themselves in their respective parts.

The visually impaired person in the coping phase may exhibit certain tendencies that need to be counteracted by the professional.

1. A self-conscious fear of failure may on occasion be a deterrent to further progress. Especially at this phase, the situation should be structured so that the visually impaired person is likely to succeed. Much time and effort are required to develop adequate coping skills; with practice comes mastery.

> First of all, fear must be trampled down—the fear of physical accidents, the fear of being unsuccessful, and the sneaking suggestion that the adventure might not be worth the effort. It would be so easy to stay safely at home. (Bretz, 1940, pp. 87-88)

2. There will be inevitable periodic reappearances of anger and frustration, which will be vented on the professional simply because of his availability. This hostility or negativism should not be taken personally unless for some reason it was deserved.

3. A common phenomenon, particularly among the recently blinded, is a fear of danger, since they find it more difficult to anticipate and thus avoid hazardous situations. The development of adequate coping skills will help the visually impaired person to handle the dangers, thus restoring his confidence.

> There is something so unnerving about being helpless to detect a source of danger and cope with it immediately, that a mishap which might scare a seeing person for only a moment is enough to leave an indelible scar on the emotional make-up of anyone who is blind. . . .
> One of the hardest things about learning to live in darkness is that one cannot see danger until it is too late, and the only thing to do is to guard against every risk as carefully as possible. (Dahl, 1962, pp. 50, 68)

4. For professionals and family members who have enjoyed being needed and wanted, the newly acquired confidence and independence of the visually impaired person may be threatening. In order to minimize possible resentments, family members should be helped to understand his desire to exercise his new freedom (Acton, 1976).

5. Since the visually impaired person is frequently self-conscious or embarrassed regarding the use of adaptive aids or techniques, the professional will want to emphasize that successful accomplishment of the task is more important than the manner by which it was accomplished. Continued hard work and practice will improve his competence, and recognition by the significant others of this improvement, along with their words of encouragement, will counteract his sense of embarrassment regarding special equipment (Mangold, 1982).

Fitting (1957) studied the factors associated with adjusting to blindness, and his findings have implications for the professional. He reported that problems were frequently related to confidence in one's ability to cope, attitudes and relationships toward sighted people, concept of self as a blind person, family relationships, attitude toward training as a method of solving problems, and occupational outlook.

From another perspective, Younie and Rusalem (1971) listed the obstacles to rehabilitation as "inability to travel, poor personal hygiene, inability to find help, unrealistic aspirations, lack of emotional stability, lack of knowledge about jobs, inadequate communication skills, lack of family support, poor work motivation, poor social behavior" (p. 21). The professional should be able to recognize these obstacles when they occur and should, where possible, structure the rehabilitation program to alleviate them or prevent them from occurring.

In addition, the professional must develop a sensitivity to the readiness of the visually inpaired person to begin the acquisition of coping skills. VanderKolk (1981) observed that—

> coping skills, or the willingness to develop these skills, are a sign that the client is at a stage where rehabilitation or education plans will be worthwhile. This is the stage where the client accepts the modified self, limitation and all, and recognizes that blindness is only one small part of herself or himself. The client focuses more on the new skills necessary to return to an active life. Brief and less intense lapses into previous states may occur, but not to the degree that they will interfere with the development of

coping skills. Thus, attitudes and action combine to form a set of coping abilities that will return the client to the family, work, or school. (p. 143)

Adjusting, adaptive or maladaptive, involves three components: the knowledge of coping—cognitive; the behaviors of coping—action; and the feelings of coping—affective. It is the latter, a person's attitudes and the way he feels while coping, that differentiates between adaptive and maladaptive coping. A person can cope with all the appropriate behaviors without necessarily any reference to or change in his sense of self-esteem, self-worth, or self-acceptance.

Within certain limits, seeking self-acceptance and self-esteem in one's successes, achievements, or competencies is a normal drive, as discussed in Chapter 5. The struggle for self-esteem frequently finds its expression in the desire to try to prove one's adequacy, competence, equality, and normalcy.

> I wanted two things from college, each with equal passion. I wanted to learn everything I could, and I wanted to prove—not only to the faculty and the students, but to myself, too—that I could compete on even terms with people who could see.... The Sisters... couldn't give me any special considerations because of my blindness. That was fair enough; the last thing I wanted was to be treated any differently from others. (Caulfield, 1960, p. 39)

Sooner or later, however, one tires of the struggle to prove oneself and finally decides to get on with the business of living. Although a contributor to self-esteem, successful performance alone through the development of adequate coping skills is insufficient to develop and maintain a positive self-esteem.

> To this day everything I do takes me longer than it would a normally sighted person. Extra work time is the lot of the partially sighted person.
> But, ultimately, effort is not the solution. . . . If my problem was blindness, then effort might be the best solution. But if my problem was the pain of loss, then effort alone would not do it. . . .
> I grew steadily more angry and frustrated because I simply could not win this battle by effort alone.
> Before an elephant can begin to dance, he must understand what he

needs to be able to dance. . . .

The point is whether or not that improved performance is where I find self-worth.

It is not. Self-worth comes not from performance but from God. I am worthy not because of what I do but because of what I am. I am a creature of the Creator. (Kemper, 1977, pp. 79, 150)

PHASE SEVEN: SELF-ACCEPTANCE AND SELF-ESTEEM

"I like me," "I am somebody"

Life is a process of adjusting and accommodating to the various physical and social demands encountered day by day. Successfully meeting the demands of life does not necessarily result in, but certainly contributes to, positive self-esteem or self-acceptance. The visually impaired person can accept the fact of blindness and its implications without accepting himself. One can learn to cope with the demands of blindness, can learn to live within the real limitation or barriers imposed by blindness, and can still have poor self-esteem. It is a travesty when one's adjusting process falls short of self-acceptance and self-esteem. Many times the individual does not even realize that it could be otherwise.

I love this new life I have fashioned for myself and whatever success I have achieved. It has helped me tremendously, but it hasn't helped me to accept my blindness. I don't think that I ever will accept it.

I don't have a very positive reaction to other blind people. I can't be too comfortable with them because I keep seeing myself in them. Those that I have seen en masse, so to speak, have been, for the most part, a very pathetic group. I've seen them at the . . . when I had a show there. Most of them were not mentally alert. If they had been sighted people, I would not have enjoyed their company. (Sperber, 1976, p. 238)

Acceptance of Blindness

Probably it would always be one thing or another. If only this, if only that. . . . But it did begin to penetrate: I couldn't see. I couldn't move easily from room to room. I would call people by the wrong names. I would have to settle for small bits of information, carefully selected. (Potok, 1980, pp. 270-271)

The acceptance of blindness and its implications is a prerequisite to self-acceptance and self-esteem. Hicks (1979) suggested that "a state of resolution is reached in which one has a full acceptance of the fact of the loss and has acquired new behavior and relationships, has extinguished nonadaptive behavior, and is rid of disruptive emotions" (p. 172). The following excerpt illustrates that the resolution or acceptance of the fact of irrevocable blindness must take place at both the intellectual and emotional levels.

> One day that light threw a searching beam which fell upon something which astonished me— it revealed to me that I had never actually accepted the fact of blindness. I had realized it, yes—but realization and acceptance, I suddenly saw, are not the same thing at all. That I had not accepted the blindness had been subtly hidden from my conscious thinking and two errors had grown out of this situation.
>
> In the first place, I must have been regarding the blindness as a temporary state—been maintaining to myself that this was an ephermeral, fleeting condition. Somewhere beneath the surface I must have been telling myself that I was just marking time—was masquerading all the while and some day the mask would come off and I would see again, and all this foolish, difficult, adjusting kind of living arrangement would be tossed aside and I could forget the whole tedious business.
>
> The second error I had been guilty of was that, although I had learned to do many things in this hampered, constricting kind of existence, I had been operating almost entirely with a sighted person's approach. . . . Both of these errors were evasion—hypocrisy, pretense, deception, insincerity—tends to wear one down, emotionally, mentally, physically. . . .
>
> I had been guilty of the worst kind of insincerity—self-deception. . . .
>
> True "acceptance" does not mean an attitude of negative resignation, a sorrowful mien, a wringing of the hands in self-pity, thereby distressing those about one. Rather, "acceptance," as I understand and use the term, means to look squarely at a troublesome situation, then to proceed from there to do whatever is possible within the framework of that situation. (McCoy, 1963, pp. 103-105)

The intellectual and emotional acceptance of the reality of blindness is still, however, insufficient for self-acceptance and self-esteem. "The person's ability to function is affected by what he feels about himself and his condition. He may make some gains through physical retraining, but if he has not resolved his feelings about what has happened to him, it is quite possible that he will not use what he has learned" (Schulz, 1980, p. 147). On the other hand, if he is only given psychological counseling without training to develop appropriate coping skills "to restore his independence and self-confidence, he can never feel that he is an adequate individual" (Schulz, 1980, p. 148).

Either consciously or unconsciously a blind person's feelings about himself may follow the illogical train of thought: "Blindness is bad; I am blind; therefore, I am bad." In the first place, not all unfortunate or unpleasant events in a person's life are necessarily "bad." While the fact of blindness must be integrated and internalized into one's self-concept, its socially derogatory and negative overtones must be confronted and dispelled rather than also being internalized. For some this distinction may be understood readily, while for others, it may take years.

It turned out to be a matter of years before blindness—hers, mine, all of ours—became, quite simply, the inability to see with our eyes, nothing more. (Potok, 1980, p. 163)

When one begins to assess some of the positive aspects of his life as a blind person, he is on the road toward making the important distinction between the fact of blindness and the socially derogatory overtones.

Blindness has taught me to face facts, to enjoy little things, to appreciate people, and to laugh at myself. (Bretz, 1940, p. 181)

There is a delicate balance between too much concern about blindness and too little, between total absorption in blindness and rejecting all blindness-related people and matters. According to Wright (1960) "to accept one's disability and oneself as a person with a disability by no means implies an all-absorbing interest in disability-connected problems. Too much pre-occupation may be as much a sign of maladjustment as ostensibly too little" (p. 47). She continued by stating that, in contrast, "accepting one's disability and oneself as a person with a disability does imply a certain feeling of kinship with others who have the disability, a feeling of knowing such a person a little even though he is a stranger" (pp. 47-48).

Cholden (1958) listed five internal forces that cause individuals to resist acceptance of blindness:

> (a) the inertia, or resistance to change of the human personality; (b) the stereotypes the patient has held relating to the blind as a class; (c) the irrational feelings concerning blindness with its sexual meanings and historical connotations as a punishment for sins; (d) the minority group aspect of blindness with its meanings in terms of inferior status and personal devaluation; (e) the necessary dependencies which accompany this handicap. (pp. 76-77)

Self-acceptance

> If someone were to come up to Bob and ask, "If you could have one wish come true, what would it be?" I'd lay odds a hundred to one that he'd say something like, "Enough money so we could afford a new car," or "Enough money so we could live in Florida and I wouldn't have to work," or something equally mercenary. It just wouldn't occur to him to say, "I'd wish I could see." (Moore, 1960, p. 131)

A self-accepting person is one who has learned to accept all of his personal attributes, the strengths along with the limitations, the assets along with the liabilities. He does not permit conceit to result from overly inflating strengths and assets, nor does he allow the limitations and liabilities to be personally devaluating. He is at peace with himself; he is comfortable with himself; he likes himself. Self-acceptance does not mean that he necessarily likes or appreciates all of his attributes. However, he recognizes that everyone possesses some perceived negative attributes or limitations that do not detract from his fundamental dignity and worth as a person. Self-love, self-approval, and self-respect are all key ingredients of self-acceptance.

> Ever since I was a young child, people have stared at me. Knots of window-shoppers are suddenly silent as I pass, and when they think me out of earshot they say, "Isn't it a shame!"
> And when someone helps me across a crowded intersection, his curiosity cannot be restrained.
> "What's it like? Just darkness, eh? Always dark like midnight, I suppose? It must be very strange. But, then, you have a sixth sense,

don't you? All you people do. Very strange!"

"Well," I asked myself, "am I so strange?"

I have come to the conclusion that they are right—I am peculiar. I am convinced, also, that those window-shoppers, if they considered the question seriously would come to the same conclusion about themselves. For we are all oddities, all peculiar, all individuals. (Russell, 1962, pp. 9-10)

Rogers (1959) differentiated between conditional and unconditional acceptance. People value and accept themselves as they are valued and accepted by others. If others' acceptance has been conditional, that is, their acceptance depends on the visually impaired person's meeting certain conditions, then his acceptance of himself is more likely to be conditional. Conditional acceptance always carries with it the possibility that a person can fail to meet the conditions, making him vulnerable to rejection by others and by himself. Unconditional acceptance, on the other hand, is acceptance not for what one does but for who one is, for the intrinsic value as a person.

To be more specific, a person who is visually impaired must see himself, first, as a person of dignity and worth and, second, as a person who, among many other attributes, happens also to be blind. To be self-accepting, a blind person does not need to like blindness but he does need to internalize blindness as one of his many characteristics. As is true of his other attributes, blindness is always present, sometimes forgotten, but nonetheless permeating all of life without dominating. He recognizes the danger of viewing sight as a condition of acceptance but instead, has found the peace, freedom, and security of unconditional self-acceptance. He no longer feels the need to struggle against blindness as an external force because he is comfortable with his internalized attributes including blindness, satisfied with his self-concept. He has learned satisfactory and socially appropriate means of meeting his own needs.

Blindness is a very real fact, and if accepted will not grow larger. It is never nonexistent; it is always present, permeates all of life without dominating. (Bretz, 1940, p. 172)

Self-esteem

The concept of self-esteem is closely related to the concept of self-acceptance. As discussed in Section II, self-esteem is the affective component of a person's self-concept, the way he feels about himself. High self-esteem is reflected in a person's judgment of his own value and worth. Individuals with high self-esteem tend, during their childhood, to have a close relationship with parents who accepted and encouraged them, who were themselves emotionally stable and self-actualized. An individual with high self-esteem tends to exhibit the intrapersonal characteristics of trust and acceptance of self, avoidance of undue worry, confidence in their own judgments, expectations of being successful, being more self-directed, and being more open to new experiences and change. He displays the interpersonal characteristics of a sensitivity to the needs of others, a feeling of value and equality with respect to others, less susceptibility to others' attempts to influence him, acceptance of criticism more readily, a tendency to take a more active and assertive role, and maintains relationships characterized by mutual feelings of respect, dignity, value and worth (see Chapter 6).

> Tom put his heavy coat over my shoulders and explained that he didn't know where he was and that it would be dangerous to sail until the fog had lifted. I tried to fathom his problem and then suggested, "Why don't you sail in the direction of the lighthouse?"
> "I can't see the light," said Tom.
> "But you can hear it." I replied, referring to the foghorn.
> Old Tom suddenly became uncharacteristically animated. "D'ya think you could guide us home, Tommy?"
> For the first time in my life I was aware of being able to do something useful and special, something that even a wise, grownup person like Tom McDonagh couldn't do. It seemed totally natural to me to point the boat toward the foghorn. (Sullivan and Gill, 1975, p. 21)

Wylie (1961), in her extensive review of the literature on self-esteem, observed that the typical studies reported a positive correlation between self-regard and personal adjustment. In other words, a healthy adjustment to life with blindness usually results in self-acceptance and self-esteem. This relationship is seen in what Giarratana-Oehler (1976) called "identity integration." "Identity integration is a state of self-actualization in which the individual has learned to live with his disability, to realize his limitations, to involve himself in a world outside of himself, and to return to the fulfillment of life goals" (p. 239). Steinzor (1966) reported the following healthy adjusting attitudes and coping skills among the blind children he studied: "the ability to recognize their handicaps and to accept them, their aspirations to find a place in a world based on sight, their ability to identify themselves as persons rather than as blind, and the strength not to gloss over differences between sightedness and blindness" (p. 311). Both of the above quotations imply that good adjustment to blindness is associated with self-acceptance and self-satisfaction within a sighted world.

> I approached life from a different angle, perhaps a selfish one. The fact that stared me in the face was that I had to live with myself. Therefore, I must make myself a companion I could live with. (Bretz, 1940, p. 67)

Acceptance of and by Others

With the newly acquired self-acceptance and self-esteem of this phase of the adjusting process, the individual is now ready to relate positively to others. "When the individual perceives and accepts into one consistent and integrated system all his sensory and visceral experiences, then he is necessarily more understanding of others and is more accepting of others as separate individuals" (Rogers, 1951, p. 520). There is a connection between the ability to love oneself and the ability to love another (Fromm, 1939). The person who feels unloved and unlovable is unable to love another (Horney, 1937). Citing twenty-one studies, Wylie (1961) concluded "on the whole evidence supports the hypothesized association between self-acceptance (or high self-regard) and acceptance of others (or high regard for others)" (p. 240).

"Acceptance is a 'two-way street,' and the blind and the sighted both have a responsibility in traveling on it"

(Routh, 1970, p. 11). Each has a responsibility to make himself acceptable, to accept himself, thus enabling each to accept the other. If the blind person is self-accepting and self-assured, then the others are more likely to accept him and his blindness in an unassuming, natural way. The converse is equally true; if the sighted person is self-accepting and self-assured, then the blind person is more likely to accept him in an unassuming, natural way.

> Chris told me he had looked ahead just in time to see the civic-minded man bounce off my bulk and land firmly on his bottom. . . .
> If the people I was working with had been unduly sympathetic or scared to mention these incidents, they probably would have worried me far more than they did. Instead they extracted all the amusement they could out of them at my expense. They took it for granted that I was blind, but they did not try to set me apart as someone to be handled with care. I felt they really accepted me as one of them. If I used a hackneyed phrase in a story or an outlandish misspelling, I heard about it as much as anyone else would. . . . I noticed many times that somebody new on the staff at first would show me just a little more politeness than usual, but slowly they would follow the tone set by the others. (Edwards, 1962, pp. 65-66)

Acceptance of oneself and acceptance of others include a responsibility to maintain a healthy relationship.

> My situation might have been much worse. It seems to me that everyone has to make adjustments to life, that we all have our limitations, but that if we are wise we do not make other people miserable by concentrating on these limitations. One of the fundamental responsibilities of every human being in his relationship with others is to create happiness, not destroy it. We also have responsibilities toward ourselves, The prime one is not to make ourselves miserable by dwelling on something we can do nothing about. . . .
> I relish life and know that there is still much for me to do and to know. (Carver, 1961, pp. 176, 208)

In contrast, if a blind person is unable to accept himself, he is unable to accept anyone else and his tendency toward ego-centric behavior is perpetuated.

> Every man has certain physical and emotional needs. If these needs are not adequately filled, the possibility of their being filled is seriously threatened or curtailed, the blind person may experience a serious maladjustment, causing him continuing problems

in human relationships. . . . If a client has no inner emotional peace and calm, and does not feel accepted, significant, and safe, he does not have good mental health. (Routh, 1970, p. 47)

A person who feels that his emotional needs are not being met, who feels that he is not accepted by others, may conclude he is unworthy and consequently may reject himself. Hamachek (1971) observed that "the self-rejecting person, if he also rejects others, is likely to be rejected by them in turn, with the inevitable consequence of reinforcing the original maladjustment" (p. 231). Just as it is true that acceptance and approval between two individuals are reciprocally and mutually reinforcing, so are mistrust, rejection, and disapproval mutually reinforcing.

Adjusting, a Continuous Process

Self-acceptance and self-esteem are not fixed qualities. If and when they are achieved, in whole or in part, they do not remain constant for the rest of life. When certain situations or events produce anxiety or doubts about one's acceptability or worthiness, one is likely to cycle back through some or all of the adjusting process. "This cycle occurs each time another implication of the loss is discovered and examined, and assumptions and behavior must be unlearned and relearned" (Hicks, 1979, p. 172). The confrontation with another trauma and the cycling back through the phases can occur at any age, by a child or an adult, and whether self-acceptance and self-esteem are recently acquired or long-standing.

> David challenged us all. He asked the why and the where and the how of all we did, and went on asking. He took his own time and made his own decisions. . . .
> David had a refrain which would have been monotonous if it had not been so gratifying. "Leave me alone, I can do it myself," varied by, "Leave me alone, I know how." . . .
> Obviously he was not going to have any great difficulty in learning to read Braille, and the satisfaction which he felt and the praises freely given helped him for quite a little time. We were less tense and anxious for him, and congratulating ourselves on his acceptance, when he dropped his little bomb. In school, suddenly and without

warning, in fact without precedence, he went into a violent temper tantrum, screaming and kicking and throwing his books, frightening all. He was almost without control and desperately unhappy. He worked out his passion and sat, empty and drained. It took endless time and talk and suggesting and loving to explain the problem and weeks to regain the confidence and pleasure he had had in school. (Lunt, 1965, pp. 56-57)

"Handicapped persons encounter more new psychological situations than do non-handicapped" (Davies, 1967, p. 116). The situation or event that precipitates another trauma and resulting adjusting behavior may or may not be related to one's immediate surroundings. Without an appropriate explanation from the individual, an observer might be totally bewildered by some uncharacteristic behaviors such as withdrawal, angry outbursts, or plaintive self-pity. The situations or events that may precipitate anxiety or doubts about one's acceptability or worthiness include—

1. new or strange physical surroundings that require the application of problem-solving abilities (finding the bathroom at a party or finding the limousine to a hotel);
2. new social environment where one's reception is uncertain (curiosity, scorn, rejection, pity or acceptance);
3. confrontation with unresolved conflict between one's perceived personal attributes and reality or between one's personal attributes and another's defining attributes (competence vs. incompetence, attractive vs. repulsive) (see Chapter 6).

After Vajda adjusted to a gradual loss of sight for eleven years, depression was precipitated by another postponement of cataract surgery.

The tornado erupted in full force within me. For more than a decade I had been building in myself a dam of discipline so as to be able to live and laugh in my gradually darkening world. Now the dam had crumbled and I was drowning in a flood of despair. (Vajda, 1974, p. 19)

The adjusting process is dynamic and fluid. One's self-acceptance and self-esteem are vulnerable to the forces at work within the individual and within one's physical and social environment. Sensitivity to the dynamic nature of the adjusting process will help explain unusual adjusting behavior and will give the opportunity to provide needed support and understanding.

Role of the Professional

During the time when the student or client is struggling with accepting the fact and implications of blindness, the professional's primary function is to provide realistic feedback within a context of warm support. Wright (1960) recommended—

> the assimilation of the negative aspects of disability within a self-concept that could remain positive. Being brought face to face for the first time with one's shortcomings in a hostile and rejecting environment can be such a devastating experience that precautions must be taken to avoid this, particularly in childhood. It makes all the difference in the world if painful facts about the self are first realized in a friendly and accepting atmosphere. In the former case there is a cementing between the self-core and the negative fact, whereas in the latter case there is a separation. (p. 161)

Care must be taken to maintain a proper attitude toward one's strengths and limitations. The blind person cannot afford to ignore completely the limitations; neither can he afford to dwell on them.

> There are things I have lost, which I have promised myself not to think about, and there are valuable and important things I have gained. (Blackhall, 1962, p. 166)

The professional can help the student or client understand that his life can be as full and as rich as he makes it. If one spends his time on the possibilities of life, his life will be full and satisfying, he won't have time to sit around and mope about the "limitations." The possibilities of life as a blind person are indeed extensive and numerous.

The defense mechanisms, such as denial, repression, and projection, are no longer necessary for the one who has accepted the fact and implications of blindness. The professional is in a position to help the student recognize the situations where he might be tempted to try concealing his blindness or try playing "as if" and help him make a conscious effort to extinguish their use. The longing for sight should be diminishing with time.

> "And you, Bill," Philippa asked, "what is it you most want—your sight?"
>
> Bill was silent for a moment. "In theory, I suppose, yes," he said, "but I never think of it that way. When I knew that I would not see again, I put all thought of sight—even as a wish—out of my mind." (Yates, 1960, p. 171)

The professional must continue to maintain a proper balance between the cognitive and affective components of the training program. Behavioral coping skills without attitudinal coping skills are insufficient to establish or reestablish self-acceptance and self-esteem. "There is a danger that one may assume that teaching a person to do everything he did prior to disability will automatically insure adjustment" (Cohn, 1961, p. 18). This principle is equally true for the socially traumatized blind person. Teachers and parents dare not focus on the development of compensatory skills at the expense of providing for the affective growth.

When the individual has acquired some sense of healthy self-acceptance and positive self-esteem, it is time for the professional to back off to permit the student or client to exercise his independence and self-confidence. Some parents along with some teachers are guilty of continuing to provide support and training far longer than necessary. Too much of a good thing is as bad as too little. In addition, there are students and clients who have developed good coping skills and who have gained a measure of self-acceptance and self-esteem but who are reluctant to assert themselves. They are the ones who need to be pushed, coaxed, cajoled, and even bribed to get out, to put forth the time and effort, to put their new skills to use.

The student will at times feel self-conscious. He may feel "different" because he is performing a task or function in a manner different from his peers. In order to overcome the negative feelings of self-consciousness, he must be convinced that "different" is not "bad" (Cohn, 1961).

> So I began to understand that there was something different about
> me, but not—because of my parents' wise tactics—that I was in any way
> inferior. (Hocken, 1977, p. 6-7)

Relatively speaking, the accomplishment of a task or
function is more important than the manner of accomplishing it. It is more important that a book be read than whether
one reads regular print, regular print with low vision aids,
large print, braille, or recordings. Blindness and its unique
ways of doing some things should not be a barrier to
achieving a sense of accomplishment.

The professional may want to warn his student or client
about the problem of maintaining a balance between
utilizing behaviors that are appropriate for the blind and
utilizing behaviors that are common to all, blind or sighted.
The blind person does not wear a sign around his neck
saying "I am blind," for that would put blindness, rather
than the person, in the focal point of attention. The
specialized aids and techniques that have become a natural
part of his life are not always in use, nor are they always
visible. The self-assured and self-confident blind person
with excellent coping skills may, at times be accused of
"faking" blindness. Frequently some humor will help bridge
the awkwardness of the moment.

> Shortly after his graduation from W.S.B., Bill showed another phase
> of adjustment one night when walking the two miles to his father's
> home. The traffic cop stopped him to ask why he did not cross the
> street in the crosswalk. When the cop could not believe his story of
> blindness, Bill promptly removed both eyes for proof. The baffled cop
> said, "Get in, I'll take you home." (Fries, 1980, p. 379)

Finally, the role of the professional is to instill in the
visually impaired person a desire and ability to continue to
grow in self-understanding, in the understanding of others,
and in problem-solving skills. If the blind person understands that an unfamiliar situation or trauma may throw
him back into some phase of the adjusting process, he is
then in a better position to understand his own feelings and
reactions as well as the feelings and reactions of others. It is
not wrong occasionally to feel those old emotions of self-

pity, anger, discouragement, and desire to withdraw. Good coping behaviors include the ability to mobilize one's resources to solve any new problems encountered.

SUMMARY

The process of adjusting to life's demands with blindness is the same process as adjusting to any severe trauma whether divorce, loss of employment, initial onset of blindness, initial awareness of social stigma of blindness, or subsequent social and physical traumas of blindness. There is no fixed state of "adjustment to blindness" but rather a continuous process of adjusting to daily demands of life with the added attribute of blindness. This adjusting process involves three components that must be carefully balanced and orchestrated: the knowledge of facts involved—cognitive; the behaviors involved—action; and the feelings involved—affective.

The seven phases described in this chapter are sequential, not hierarchical; they are overlapping, not distinct. A majority of the individuals adjusting to a severe trauma experience, to one degree or another, most if not all of the phases described. A person may begin progressing through the phases but at some point in the process may find that he is unable or unwilling to continue any further. Unfortunately, he may remain in this phase indefinitely. Every time a person confronts another trauma (an unresolved discrepancy or an unfamiliar situation), he may cycle back through some or all of the adjusting phases before regaining some measure of self-acceptance and self-esteem.

Adjusting with blindness is more than mourning and succumbing, more than a reaffirmation of life, more than learning new behavioral and attitudinal coping skills. Adjusting with blindness is less than satisfactory until the individual reaches the potential of self-acceptance and self-esteem as a person, first of all, and then as a person who happens to be blind.

Self-acceptance is the ability to like oneself amidst all the perceived positive and negative qualities or personal attributes. Self-esteem is the judgment that one is worthy. Unfortunately, self-acceptance and self-esteem are too frequently based on reflections from others (Chapter 4), successful performance (Chapter 5), and the ability to achieve intra- and interpersonal harmony by resolving discrepancies (Chapter 6) rather than simply on the intrinsic value of being a person, a part of God's creation. The more the visually impaired individual depends on reflected appraisals and successful performances for self-acceptance and self-esteem, the less stable he is apt to be in the face of the many traumas of blindness.

Figure 13 summarizes the dynamic and fluid nature of the process as well as the potential for maladjustment at any phase in the process.

Although the adjusting model provides a general framework for conceptualizing the process, each person responds to trauma quite individualistically. Each brings to the trauma his own unique personality, his own unique set of personal attributes, his own already developed set of coping behaviors. The significance of the trauma is interpreted differently by each depending on his set of goals, values, and standards. The intensity and duration of each phase of the adjusting process will vary from one person to the next, from one time to the next, depending on the various factors outlined in the next chapter.

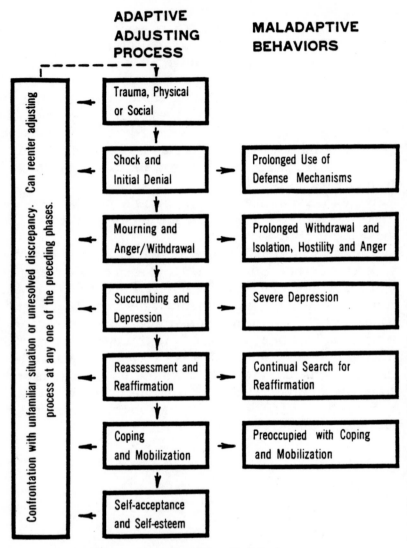

Figure 13. Adjusting with Blindness

Chapter 9

FACTORS INFLUENCING
THE ADJUSTING PROCESS

Most persons traumatized by either the initial onset of blindness or the confrontation with the social stigma of blindness experience, to one degree or another, the phases of the dynamic and continual adjusting process described in the last chapter. However, there is considerable variability among blind individuals with respect to the intensity and duration of their cognitive, behavioral, and emotional reactions in each phase. This chapter is devoted to identifying some of the factors that influence the adjusting process and that contribute to the variability among traumatized persons. Some of these factors, such as age and intelligence, are characteristics the individual himself brings to the trauma. Other factors, such as support network and resources, are defined by a person's physical and social environment (Blank, 1957; Moos and Tsu, 1977; Neu, 1975). Since one of the most critical factors is the individual's desire for and drive toward independence, the chapter concludes with a discussion of the dependence-independence continuum and the relationship between desired independence and required assistance.

FACTORS INTERNAL TO THE INDIVIDUAL

Personality Characteristics

The personality (including ego strengths and self-concept)

established prior to the trauma is one of the most significant predictors of the outcome of the adjusting process (Blank, 1957; Cholden, 1958; Dover, 1959; Emerson, 1981; Rusalem, 1972; VanderKolk, 1981). This principle is equally true whether the trauma is the recent onset of blindness or the recent confrontation with the social stigma of blindness. In either case, the personality and ego strength the individual brings to the crisis will determine, in large measure, the nature of the outcome. The personality characteristics demonstrated in the following excerpt were developed prior to the crisis.

> I had accepted blindness and thought myself cognizant of its limitations. Well, I wasn't. In every picayune daily action, blindness lurked to trip me up. It was amazing and it was constant. I didn't get mad, but I did get fiercely determined to win the fight or go down with flag flying. . . .
> I dug away the sand of discouragement shovelful by shovelful. Sometimes the shovel wasn't really full, but persistent effort finally found the rock of courage. Courage has been a firm foundation stone, for when the winds of adversity have whipped up a gale, my little house has stood solid. (Bretz, 1940, pp. 68, 189)

After testing 114 recently blinded adults and a significant other for each subject, Greenough et al. (1978) discovered that those experiencing less depression had been viewed as "assertive, independent, stubborn, venturesome, uninhibited, experimenting, free-thinking, aggressive, and socially bold" (p. 87) prior to their loss of vision, while those experiencing more severe depression had been viewed as "humble, mild, obedient, conforming, shy, restrained, conservative" (p. 87). It is logical to assume that research will someday demonstrate that similar patterns emerge among the congenitally blind in their reactions to personal and social traumas. In a closely related field, a study of personality characteristics among physically handicapped children related quality of adjustment to "aggressiveness, attentiveness, self-control, friendliness, emotional stability, cooperation, tolerance, cheerfulness, effort, sensitivity, and anxiety" and concluded that "strong dependency needs are more characteristic of well-adjusted than poorly-adjusted handicapped children" (Mussen and Newman, 1958, p. 278). A willingness to admit realistic dependency needs, while maintaining a basic desire for and drive toward independence, is associated with a more effective adjusting process.

Similarly, VanderKolk's (1981) discussion of the personality determinants of adjustment among the recently blinded may apply equally well to the congenitally blind.

A somewhat dependent person will likely become more dependent. A very independent person may at first feel a greater shock, and perhaps depression, then assert his or her independence to the maximum extent possible. Those who overreacted to the stresses of everyday life are more likely to suffer a great deal emotionally when they lose their vision. The socially introverted person may become a recluse. (p. 142)

A person's sense of humor is another critical determiner of the quality of the adjusting process (Schulz, 1980). Humor can serve to break the awkward tension occasionally felt by the sighted. The ability to laugh at oneself, to laugh at the ridiculousness and the incongruities of life, is both an indicator and a facilitator of good adjusting.

"I ran into a blind man!" he gasped. "I was walking up to catch the streetcar and thinking about having to cross that damnable Grand Avenue. I had my cane across my arm and was listening for traffic, and bang! I ran into someone and damn near went down. The thought flashed through my mind, why the devil doesn't he watch where he's going! and I grabbed at him, and my hand touched a cane, and just then Audrey said something, and I recognized him! He had just made it across Grand Avenue and was feeling so set up about doing it unscathed, that he wasn't using his cane either. It drew blood on both of us."
Both of us almost collapsed, we laughed so hard. (Moore, 1960, pp. 169-170)

The evening was most enjoyable, with very interesting people, some of whom I had never met before. I came home happy and excited, for it was good to know that it didn't seem to make any difference to those present that I couldn't see. . . . [Then she realized she had gone out with one white shoe and one black shoe on.]
I was on the verge of tears. Instead, I suddenly started to laugh. I sat down and laughed and laughed. If I were to take every mistake I made

as a tragedy, I would ruin every good time I had. I would always be worrying and there would be no sense in that. (Dahl, 1962, pp. 103-104)

However, not all expressions of humor are indicators of healthy adjusting (Schulz, 1980). Humor that is self-derogatory may be an indicator of poor self-esteem. A light, flippant reaction to the trauma of blindness may be an avoidance or denial mechanism that directs attention away from a sensitive issue. Humor that is expressed in ridicule or sarcasm is frequently masking hostility and anger.

Prior Coping Experiences

Along with the basic personality characteristics, previous experiences with traumas or crises help to establish a person's style of coping and pattern of problem solving (Emerson, 1981). "The way the individual has learned to cope with his major life problems and emergencies antedating his blindness will largely determine his ego-recovery capacity as far as blindness is concerned, assuming, of course that the external obstacles are not too great" (Cholden, 1958, p. 73). The congenitally blind youth who encounters personal or social trauma in high school or adulthood has already established his adaptive behaviors from prior coping experiences.

Prior Attitudes Toward Blindness

The pretrauma attitudes toward blindness influence a person's adjusting process. For the recently blinded, these attitudes are more detached and abstract since they are usually developed long before the actual onset of blindness. On the other hand, the pretrauma attitudes of the congenitally blind are much more personalized as they are referring to one of his own personal attributes. In either case these pretrauma attitudes are predominantly negative, derogatory, and devaluating (see Chapter 3).

These attitudes toward blindness are usually learned unconsciously and incidentally from the significant others in one's social environment. The following excerpts illustrate the wide variability of possible sources of these attitudes. As a boy Fries developed his attitudes toward blindness by listening to his father tell about a blind grandfather.

> Why had I feared blindness? Was it because I had heard Papa tell about leading his blind father and because I had been called "Blindy" at North Starr School? After this momentous afternoon with Lyle, I felt it really would not be so bad to be blind, as I had feared so long. It isn't how much we can see but the way we meet our handicap that counts. (Fries, 1980, p. 86)

Some of the negative stereotypic attitudes about blind persons were adopted by Mitchell apparently unconsciously and perhaps intuitively.

> The indignation I recognized fairly soon, for was it not natural? Why should I, through no fault of my own, be forced to contend with such difficulties? But it took me a very much longer time to track down and admit the other emotion, for it turned out to be not particularly praiseworthy, to be in fact an intense reluctance to find myself on a par with people whom I had always regarded chiefly as objects of pity, and therefore living on a lower plane than myself. It galled me to think that I was now one of these inadequate beings, could not hope to live on equal terms with the rest of the world, had been pushed into a position of inferiority. I was wrong of course. I made the mistake of confusing inequality with inferiority. (Mitchell, 1964, p. 28)

The source for the negative attitude in the following anecdote was the posters made by the peers, totally dominating any possible positive impact of the excellent lecture. As so often happens, the negative overshadowed the positive.

> I knew of this anxiety only that it was inseparably connected with my feelings about the Seeing Eye. From the moment, several months before, when the idea of obtaining a dog had first been suggested to me, I had felt a certain distaste for the place. I had been reluctant to believe in the permanence of my blindness and shrank from accepting so public and concrete a badge of handicap as a cripple might shrink from the first sight of a corrective shoe. In recalling a lecture given by Morris Frank, the owner of the first Seeing Eye dog, when I had been a student at The Hill School, I remembered, not the gay and confident presence of Mr. Frank, but the posters which had heralded his appearance. Drawn by the art students, they depicted blind men and women being led by their dogs in a style which combined adolescent literalism with the motionless unreality of an Egyptian tomb fresco. My

vanity was grated by the mere thought of identifying myself with those stiffened profiles. (Putnam, 1952, p. 20)

Regardless of the source, devaluating pretrauma attitudes impact negatively on a person's adjusting process. The more negative the pretrauma attitudes are toward blindness, the more severe is the trauma and the more difficult is the adjusting process.

Intelligence

A person's intelligence is another factor influencing the adjusting process (Bauman, 1954a; Moos and Tsu, 1977). Much of the adjusting process requires problem-solving abilities. Understanding oneself and others, the recognition of the problem, the search for alternative solutions and the implementation of the best solution are all abilities associated with intelligence. As a general rule, the more intelligent a person is, the better problem-solver he is likely to be.

Bill had always liked to work out problems, mathematical ones especially. Blindness was an intriguing problem, and as he found the solution to some of its difficult aspects he began to handle himself with an ease that looked like emancipation from blindness. (Yates, 1960, p. 65)

Age at Time of Trauma

The severity of the trauma of blindness, whether the initial onset of blindness or subsequent personal and social confrontation with the stigma of blindness, is, in part, a function of the person's age. Each age has its own cluster of concerns: during birth and infancy, the development of trust and love relationships, physical and motor development; during childhood, cognitive and social development, play skills; during adolescence, search for identity and independence, preparation for career; during working years, competence and adequacy, providing for self and family; during retirement, maintaining health through declining years, less flexible pattern of behavior, loss of sensory and mental abilities, decreasing stamina.

In addition to the other factors being considered, the

severity and duration of the adjusting phases are, therefore, a function of the interaction between the initial loss of vision or the other traumas of blindness and the age-typical concern and need. "The older the child when the loss of sight occurs, the greater will be the emotional and physical impact, the longer he will take to adjust to living with impaired vision, and the more support he will need from his family" (Scott, 1977, p. 13).

There are some who argue that being blind from infancy is easier since he does not need to learn to live with a new condition, he needs only to learn to live with others' reactions to his condition. He incorporates blindness quite naturally into his set of personal attributes. He does not need to change his body image or self-concept.

> It was good that I lost my sight when I did, because having no memories of seeing, there was nothing to look back to, nothing to miss. (Mehta, 1947, p. 4)

Children are resilient and pliable. They accommodate and adapt to the stresses of life much more easily than adults. Frequently their expressed reactions to trauma seem frivolous and superficial to the adult observer.

> I began to cry, not in fear of the hospital but in fear of being separated from my parents. I remember that the doctor's secretary had her arm in a sling and after a few minutes I asked her what was wrong with her arm. For years later she marveled and reminded me of that incident, always saying that I was such a brave and generous boy for thinking of her injury at a moment when I had so many troubles of my own. I really appreciate her sentiment, but what the incident really illustrates is the limited and easily distractable attention of an eight-year-old....
> One of my first reactions to being blind was glee. I don't have to wear glasses anymore. (Hartman and Asbell, 1978, pp.25-30)

According to Lowenfeld (1971a), the concerns and needs of adolescents are compounded by blindness, especially in the areas of "sex curiosity, dating, the lure of the car, and concern for the future" (p. 184). If the trauma "occurred close to the period of adolescence, both blind child and family would probably have greater need for highly skilled help" (Abel, 1961, p. 104). The uneasy, restive, disquieting years of adolescence become even more so with blindness.

> However, except for the dances and dance lessons, I look back on
> my high school days as a kind of Dark Ages. Nothing at school had any
> relevance for me. Everything about it — the teachers, the classwork,
> the other students — all seemed remote. Part of it, I think was
> boarding with older people, being away from home and not having
> anyone who cared — or so it seemed. I am sure, too, that part of it was
> trying to find some identity in the maelstrom of five thousand
> students. It was as though I were in some shadowy world, half-awake,
> going through programmed routines, I felt adrift, lost, terribly alone
> most of the time. This wasn't such a safe world, after all. You could
> have a glorious childhood — friends, a running streak of luck — and
> then be left to go it alone.
> From the beginning of my senior year I felt a gnawing concern
> about the future. ...
> Certainly no one in the family could advise me. (Resnick, 1975, p. 54)

The trauma of blindness occurring during the working
years undermines a person's self-confidence and sense of
competence and adequacy. Frequently, it is assumed that
one can no longer continue on one's vocation, precipating
anxiety about future employment and financial independence. The severity and duration of the adjusting phases
increase with increasing number of dependents.

The older a person is, the more difficult it is to adjust or
accommodate to the trauma of blindness. Learning new
adjusting behaviors and coping skills is extremely discouraging and depressing, especially for the one whose
pattern of behavior has become rather rigid and inflexible.
Attempting to cope with the severe trauma of blindness can
be a fearful and unnerving experience especially when the
elderly are already coping with other traumas of loss of
strength, health, friends (through death), etc. In addition to
adjusting with blindness, Bretz was weak from surgery and
thyroid complications.

> It was three months after I returned home from the hospital before I
> was able to sit up at the dining table, and, when I did, I found that I had
> to sit in an armchair, not for support, but because of a strange new
> fear. Sitting in a straight chair, the space about me seemed so vast that I
> was terrorized by the thought that an unwary movement might
> plunge me headlong into it. My horror was reminiscent of the Thing

that had crouched on my hospital bed. I had to fight hard to conquer that fear — the fear of the unseeable. (Bretz, 1940, p. 43)

Degree of Vision

The amount of vision a visually impaired person has can vary from a mild loss of acuity or field of vision to low vision, to light perception, to total blindness. Persons with a severe visual loss are confronted with a reality that is undeniable, inescapable, demanding accommodation. In contrast, there are visually impaired children whose visual loss is not detected until they experience difficulties in school.

> "You have weak eyes. From now on this will be your desk."
> The following Sunday she visited our home to discuss my sight condition and advised that I have my eyes examined. This came as a surprise, for she was the first one to report that I did not see well. Neither family member nor neighbor had ever mentioned my poor vision. (Fries, 1980, p. 40)

Although not entirely conclusive, there is some evidence to support the contention that individuals at either end of the continuum of visual loss have an easier time of the adjusting process than do those in the middle (Bauman, 1964; Cowen et al., 1961; Davis, 1964). After administering the Adolescent Emotional Factors Inventory to 150 youth in residential schools for the blind and a comparable number in public schools, Bauman (1964) concluded that partially seeing students demonstrated significantly more anxiety and insecurity than did the blind students. The low vision students were characterized by such phrases as "less good adjustment," "greater sense of tension," "worry more about health," "more suspicious," "less able to meet demands of family and school," and "lack of self confidence" (p. 105). Referring to the difficulties encountered by partially seeing children, Davis (1964) suggested that "although the process of establishing a stable concept of themselves takes a longer time than it does for seeing or for blind children, by the time they have reached adulthood, the majority of this group have worked out a satisfactory resolution of a single, functional self-concept" (p. 51).

The individuals with mild visual loss, sometimes referred to as "high partials," require fewer and less extreme adaptive behaviors and skills while the totally blind require many more. Low vision persons frequently find themselves in limbo. On the one hand, they tend to reject or are unable to profit fully from the adaptive behaviors and skills that symbolize or are associated with "blindness." At the same time, they are unable to function fully independently without some basic accommodations. This ambiguous state of affairs results in a poorly defined self-concept and socially awkward situations.

> We move to an undersea setting. This one is called the Foggy Snorkel. Go into crowded room, many well-known, even good friends, all weeds and corals now until a few inches away, rather pretty. "What's she gotten so uppity about?" Do you hear it or just think you do? Can't go around explaining. If all there were to go on about their ailments—!One woman is doing so. . . . People murmur sympathy, edge away. . . .
>
> You radiate affectionate warmth on a high-gloss thin-brained male stranger, much as a mallet might come down on a box of peanut brittle. Both smiles crumble loudly; an animosity is born. "Oh excuse me, I thought you were . . ." Then a worse kind of mistake, just from too much swimming, or fear of morays among the rocks. You ask Doris, a foot away and familiar for years, if Joe is there too. "Joe?" She decomposes; . . . She not only isn't and doesn't much resemble Doris; they don't even like each other. . . .
>
> You smile sheepishly and flee, promising to explain some other time, which of course you won't even if the subtle rift doesn't grow to a permanent crevasse. (Clark, 1977, pp. 239-242).

"The more an individual has a chance to hide his disability, or the more the resulting limitations are diffused and maldefined, the more he tends to avoid integrating the necessary changes into his body image and self concept" (Safilios-Rothschild, 1970, p. 96). Unfortunately, low vision provides the individual with the opportunity to hide his disability, to play "as if" he were fully sighted. Furthermore, the limitations of low vision are more "diffused and maldefined" and therefore less well understood by the individual himself, by the significant others and by the general public.

During my (partially) seeing days, it had taken all the wits I possessed and a great deal of subterfuge to give the impression that I could see almost as well as anyone else. For I wanted so much not be thought different from other people. Now pretense was no longer possible, and yet never in my life had I longed so passionately to be like the rest of my fellow human beings. (Dahl, 1962, p. 131)

Wright (1960) provided a description of this ambiguous position of the low vision person that can only result in poor self-acceptance.

Concealing the disability does not irradicate it; it still remains in the eye of the person as the barrier to his acceptance by the sought-for group. The stigma of disability that prompts his efforts to cover up at the same time negates his efforts. Not accepting the truth, he has to pay the consequence of being in the ambiguous position of the marginal man who belongs fully to no group. Like the man without a country, he will wander in his search for acceptance that can not be his until he accepts himself. (p. 40)

Stability of Vision

The stability or constancy of vision regardless of the degree of visual loss is yet another factor influencing the adjusting process. Some conditions are stable or constant for most of one's life, some losses degenerate slowly over a period of months and even years, and still others fluctuate from one day to another and from one situation to another. Uncertainty about one's vision is frequently accompanied by anxiety and fear, keeping one's feelings in a state of flux (Schulz, 1980). Referring to the instability of vision among their patients, Oehler-Giarratana and Fitzgerald (1980) commented "for most of the patients, loss of vision would have been a relief after months and years of fluctuating vision" (p.464).

The surprising factor is that its constancy — every time I look at anything I am consciously aware of the absence of normal vision — makes it comfortable for me. If I were to have days of normal vision and days of visual loss, that would be unbearable. But the fact that it is permanent, irreparable, and irreversible, dread words when I first heard them, makes it now manageable. (Kemper, 1977, p. 102)

A person with gradually deteriorating vision may not

experience shock and depression or other phases of the adjusting process until the loss is severe enough to interfere with daily functioning. Subsequent cycles back through the adjustment process may occur with each succeeding degree of significant sight loss that requires new adaptive behavior and skills. "An individual with diabetic retinopathy enters the first stage of grieving, that of shock and denial, and remains in this stage until he becomes legally blind or very close to it. With legal blindness, his vision is sufficiently impaired for him to believe the diagnosis, and it is then that the anger and depression of grieving set in" (Giarratana-Oehler, 1976, p. 237). Persons with gradually deteriorating vision experience psychological adjusting problems, in varying degrees of intensity, with each new degree of visual loss (Stogner, 1980).

The adjusting process remains fluid when the degree of vision fluctuates from day to day and from situation to situation. Some individuals can perform some visual tasks on certain days or certain times of the day or with certain lighting conditions but be unable to perform the same task at another time. The lack of stability in vision creates additional adjusting problems.

> I notice, with surprise, that I see a good deal better at breakfast-time, not every day but usually. With my fancy light can even read a few lines of newsprint then, laboriously but still; later in the day can't even get headlines. Some days I forget for a minute or two even to be thrilled by it, get interested and read a paragraph as if none of this had happened and force of habit were still operative. Then I remember and have to guard against crazy hope. It comes, you can't help it.
> ... Fight this wild breakfast-time joy; you know it's insane; will bring you nothing but worse misery. (Clark, 1977, pp. 265-266)

Additional Complications

Another factor influencing the adjusting process is the extent to which the blind person may also be contending with additional complications that precipitate other traumas of their own, making the adjusting process more difficult. This double jeopardy results when two conditions occur simultaneously, each making the person vulnerable to discriminatory action or to being stigmatized. A blind person whose face is disfigured, a blind person who is a quadraplegic, or a blind person who is a member of a racial minority group are all potentially in double jeopardy. With each additional complication, the phases of the adjusting process become even that much more severe and intense.

Some evidence for the additional difficulties of those experiencing multiple complications was provided in a study by Barron (1971). The adjusting process of twenty blind persons who were experiencing the additional health problems of diabetes was compared with that of twenty blind from retinitis pigmentosa. Barron (1971) found that the diabetics were "more passive, depressed, docile, compliant, withdrawn and hysterical," and had "greater feelings of inadequacy and more repressed hostility and guilt. . . . They adjusted more poorly to blindness. Although they verbally deny limitations, their behavior reveals underachievement, a focus on death and resistance to emotional well-being" (p. 2296). In contrast, those with retinitis pigmentosa were found to be "more achievement oriented, aggressive, and compulsive, externalized and overcompensated" (p. 2296). Barron reported that they were better adjusted and actively searched out ways of coping with their environment.

Smithdas (1975), who is both deaf and blind, enumerated some of the additional difficulties encountered by the deaf-blind. Although they have the same need for love, acceptance, and esteem, deaf-blind persons are frequently isolated and lonely because they are ignored. The identity crisis for the deaf-blind is more ambiguous for they are able to identify fully with neither the sighted, the blind, nor the deaf. "Socially the deaf-blind belong to the deaf group, as they use the same communication methods as the deaf; but technically they belong to the blind group, because they use the tools, devices and aids, and many of the methods used by blind persons" (Smithdas, 1975, p. 3). These dual handicaps produce additional communication barriers that impede normal social development and interaction. "Many deaf-blind persons are extremely self-centered, even selfish, because they are most conscious of their own immediate wants and needs. . . . Because of their inverted awareness of their personal needs, they find it difficult to recognize the problems of others with whom they associate" (Smithdas, 1975, pp. 1-2). The addition of the complication of deafness to blindness is not simply the sum of the implications of the two independent disabilities. Rather, the double jeopardy results in a compounding and aggregating of the implications, one upon the other.

Philosophy of Life and Basic Beliefs

Why do I climb mountains? Quite simply because the mountains and I had to meet. I go for my pleasure and to conquer myself. I know of nothing more deadly than inaction, whether physical or mental. One needs to try one's strength and one's willpower, to triumph over one's destiny, to remake oneself, to put one's muscles to use. (Richard, 1966, p. 17)

Certainly, a person's philosophy of life, basic beliefs and values, and his religious faith all contribute to the quality of the adjusting process. Whether a blind person's outlook on life is basically optimistic or pessimistic influences the adjusting dynamics. Some look upon life as a game to be played and won, while others see themselves as hapless victims of life's tragedies.

According to Needham and Ehmer (1980) "Many persons who are not coping with or adjusting to their disabilities in a positive or productive manner have irrational and self-limiting belief statements about blindness" (p. 58). These more poorly adjusted individuals maintained beliefs that centered around the concepts that the value and self-worth of blind individuals varied from that of the sighted, that the blind are unique psychologically, that the blind have a special place in society, and that blindness endows magical qualities. Even though these belief statements are obviously erroneous, for the one who believes them, they impact on his adjusting process.

A person's faith in the goodness of God and in the

purposefulness of life's experiences including blindness further contributes to a more positive outcome. As discussed in Chapter 8, a dynamic faith does not emerge from a crisis, but sustains a person through that crisis.

> If she had anything to cling to during those dark days, it was the rock of her religion. Eunice never lost the belief that there had to be some purpose in her handicap. She never lost the belief that it was up to her to discover and fulfill that purpose. (Sperber, 1976, p. 75)

> The concept of a Heavenly Father being more cruel than a human father is repugnant to me. I do not blame God for my blindness.... God helps me, as my Father. (Bretz, 1940, p. 196)

FACTORS EXTERNAL TO THE INDIVIDUAL
The Role of the Physician

Frequently, an individual learns from his ophthalmologist or family physician that he has just lost or is in the process of losing his vision. The early exchange between doctor and patient tends to set the tone for the patient's future adjustment to blindness. While being sensitive and compassionate, the doctor can and should be candid and accurate. The overriding message should "point to hope for a full life, and not to hope for recovery" (Schulz, 1980, p. 151).

> Dr. Randolph had faced the hard duty of giving me the facts like a man, which was exactly the correct way. He was gentle about it, cold and matter-of-fact though his language had been. His was an excellent example. (Boswell, 1969, p. 102)

Under certain circumstances, as in the case when sight loss is gradual, the advanced preparation of the patient by physician and family should be encouraged, so that "the phase of depersonalization is eliminated and the depressive phase reduced in severity because part of the work of mourning has been accomplished in advance" (Blank, 1957, p. 12).

The ophthalmologist or family physician must be prepared to make appropriate referrals to special education and rehabilitation services within the patient's community.

Key resources and services in any community can be identified by contacting one of the following: director of special education for the local school district, the state department of education consultant for the visually handicapped, or the state vocational rehabilitation office for a vocational counselor or rehabilitation teacher.

Unfortunately, there are some ophthalmologists who have a difficult time dealing with their patients who are blind or are losing their vision.

> These two doctors were both very quiet, very precise men who were engaged in research. They never said anything about the prognosis of my case. One of them would examine me and say, "You're fine. See me next year." (Sperber, 1976, p. 29)

Cholden described the paradox:

> In his choice of ophthalmology, the doctor has already indicated a special interest in sight. This must include an interest in the conservation of sight, the importance of sight, and a need to work for the preservation of sight. . . . Blindness may be seen by the doctor as a failure of his own ability, or as a loss of his self-esteem, or as an injury to his reputation. . . . The doctor feels blindness to be such a terrible calamity that he cannot bear his own pain in breaking the news to the patient. Yet, as a result of this failure, the patient may direct against the doctor all of the hostility and anger that he feels toward fate for making him blind. (Cholden, 1958, p. 22)

> I am speaking of the doctor's inability to accept failure. We, with unhealed eyes, are an embarrassment to those who heal eyes. That is the sinister motive I harbor about doctors: They are afraid to fail. (Kemper, 1977, p. 59)

In the foreward to the book *How Does It Feel To Be Blind* (Schulz, 1980), Dr. Sherwin Sloan, M.D., associate clinical professor of ophthalmology, UCLA School of Medicine, wrote "to the ophthalmologist, the blindness of a patient may be equivalent to the death of an internist's patient. Indeed, blindness is ophthalmic death. This is why it is difficult for many ophthalmologists, optometrists, or other professionals dealing with visually handicapped patients to continue to care for these patients once they become blind." This view of blindness of "ophthalmic death" simply perpetuates a mythical, morbid association that all but destroys any potential for a positive adjustment for the blind person.

The Personal Support Network

Parents, spouses, siblings, and friends are all members of one's personal support network. Whether they like it or not, family and friends become absorbed in an adjusting process of their own. "Family adjustment is already in the rehabilitation plan—whether we want it there or not. But the *kind* of adjustment is something we may be able to influence.... Everyone, at all times, is doing the best kind of adjusting he knows how. It may be inefficient, ineffective, or even self-destructive—but it's the best that person can do at that moment" (Dishart, 1964, p. 292).

As the visually impaired individual is adjusting to the many traumas of blindness, so too are all those close to him experiencing a similar adjusting pattern (Gardner, 1982; Neu, 1975; Schulz, 1980; Scott, 1977). "Family members and friends, as well as patients, are affected by the crisis, encounter many of the same or closely related adaptive tasks, and use the same coping skills" (Moos and Tsu, 1977, p. 8).

> A few years ago, in clearing out the attic just before moving into an apartment in New York City, Mother came across my baby book. I believe that that book expresses the agony that my parents felt, far more eloquently that I ever could.
>
> The first several pages contained the usual material which fills a baby book. The date of my arrival home, the date when I got my first tooth, and so on. Suddenly, we came to a page dated May 23, 1945. It said, "We have just returned home from Boston with Harold. My baby is blind." The remaining pages were blank.
>
> The last entry in my baby book was a stark dramatic statement which reflected a stark dramatic crisis in the lives of my young parents. The prospect of a blind child, bringing with it overwhelming responsibility and burdens seemed insupportable—robbing them prematurely of their youth, their gaiety, and their freedom. (Krents, 1972, pp. 27-28)

Parents, upon learning that their infant is blind, experience severe crises in their own personal lives, and the process of coping with these crises impacts on the relationship of the parents to each other and to their growing infant. "The parents' emotional reactions to the infant's blindness may interfere with their relationship with him, especially when feelings of guilt, self-recrimination, and anxiety overwhelm them" (Cook-Clampert, 1981, p. 235). After studying 143 blind adolescents and their parents, Sommers (1944) identified five parental reactions: realistic acceptance, denial, maternal overprotection, disguised rejection, and overt rejection. In contrast, Eisenstadt (1955) has suggested that parents adjusting to blindness and their blind children experience more of a dynamic process characterized by the following stages: (1) shock and grief, during which there is an intense feeling of loss, sorrow, and disbelief; (2) bewilderment and helplessness, during which despondency usually yields to the practical question, "What do we do about it?"; (3) fears resulting from incomplete information and ambiguous statements intended to reassure; and (4) tension resulting from anxiety regarding the child's future.

Cowen et al. (1961) found a strong relationship between maternal understanding and their adolescent blind child's adjustment. Coopersmith (1967), after studying the relationship between preadolescent sighted boys and their parents, found that high self-esteem among the children was associated with parental acceptance of their children, well established limits that were enforced, and respect for freedom of expression within the defined limits. Generalizing these principles to other family members, it is possible that understanding, acceptance, and respect whether from parents, spouse, siblings, or close friends contributes greatly to a person's healthy adjustment and positive self-esteem.

Support from family and friends can be expressed in a number of ways. As illustrated by Dahl's mother, this support was demonstrated through encouragement, praise, and a sense of pride in her daughter.

> What would she have thought of me as I struggled along from one attempt to another in this new way of living? She would not have pitied me, I was sure of that. She would have encouraged me to go

ahead. And she would have found something to praise in each accomplishment, no matter how clumsily I had done it. . . .

I had thought that I hadn't done anything all day of which I could be proud. But perhaps she would have been proud of me, at least for trying. (Dahl, 1962, pp. 48-49)

Frequently, members of the support network with good intentions are tempted to provide too much support. Yates wisely recognized that the most effective support for her blind spouse was to permit him to accomplish tasks on his own and to provide assistance only when asked.

Bill's first need was to gain self-confidence. This was achieved, to an extent, as he learned to find his way in familiar surroundings, doing the things he had long been doing. Often I reached out to shield him, to assume burdens he would ordinarily have borne; but I learned to let him do things for himself, to hold back my hand until he asked for help, and to keep him seeing inwardly. (Yates, 1960, p. 65)

Unfortunately, negative attitudes and devaluating concerns of family members and friends can also be communicated consciously or unconsciously. Increased anxiety over blindness within members of the support network tends to increase the anxiety level in the blind individual (Schulz, 1980). Sommers (1944) found that parental dissatisfaction centered around blindness as a symbol of divine disfavor or personal disgrace, society's suspicion of parental disease, and guilt over deviation from social norms. The meaning given to blindness will determine the severity of the trauma experienced by the members of the support network, which, in turn, influences the severity of the trauma experienced by the blind individual.

Members of the support network experience the same phases of the adjusting process described in the previous chapter. Just as with the blind individual's adjusting process, a parent or spouse may experience some of these phases without reaching acceptance. The adjusting process for members of the support network may be just as fluid as for the blind individual when they respond to new traumas of their own.

The characteristics previously described as factors internal to the blind individual can be reexamined as additional factors internal to members of the support network. Personality, prior coping experiences, prior attitudes toward blindness, intelligence, age, and philosophy of life that members of the support network bring to the trauma also impact on the quality of the adjusting process.

Members of the support network must learn to maintain a proper balance with their other responsibilities and continue to cultivate relationships with their own support network. When a blind individual is inserted into a constellation of significant others, the blind person may require a disproportionate amount of time and effort for some activities and during certain growth periods. One of the keys to maintaining good mental health is to achieve a proper balance of time and effort among the variety of responsibilities.

> In some ways of course, Elizabeth is bound to be "special." She takes more of my time, more conscious planning for and "teaching." Yet one of the important things she must learn is to fit into a family and to understand that there are others all around her who have desires and rights. (Ulrich, 1972, p. 45)

Reactions among members of his prior support network to the visually impaired person's trauma may vary from supportive and understanding to revulsion and withdrawal. The responses of these significant others will affect how the visually impaired person responds to the trauma. Depending on the other's reactions, there may be a need for changing the composition of the support network. These significant others may react to the visually impaired person's trauma in one of the following ways:

1. Willingness to work through the value changes and the development of coping behaviors together with the traumatized person;
2. Recognition that some changes are inevitable but, for reasons of denial or unwillingness to help with the change process, tend to withdraw until changes are accomplished;
3. Refusal to recognize that the adjusting process requires

time, resulting in intolerance exhibited through unrealistic demands or unfair judgments;

4. Expectation that nothing has changed, therefore former values and behaviors continue to be utilized.

Professional Resources and Services

Timely and appropriate professional resources and services facilitate one's adjusting process. Without resources and services, the intensity and duration of the adjusting phases become more serious. Rusalem (1972) indicated that without early intervention by the professional, the newly blinded individual may fixate in one or another of the adjusting phases, thereby retarding his personal and vocational rehabilitation. He stressed that "by re-establishing earning potential while vocational self-perceptions still are amenable to vocational rehabilitation services, professional workers can preserve self-regard" (p. 21).

To be timely and appropriate, the resources and services must be available and be made known through an effective referral system. In the first of the next two excerpts, lack of professional resources and services threatened normal growth and development, while in the second, they provided a sense of adequacy and higher self-esteem.

I once visited a teenager who suffered a dynamite accident which destroyed his one eye and seriously injured the other. Neither he nor his parents had the benefit of assistance from a rehabilitation counselor nor from anyone familiar with work for the blind. The family had me stay for dinner but the son ate by himself in the kitchen. Judging by the general conversation, I felt certain that Julius ate with fingers and did not feel comfortable at the table with company. While attending W.S.B. he learned to eat skillfully and in time became socially adept. (Fries, 1980, p. 379)

My parents brought a huge upright typewriter into school, and day by day I slowly learned to type by the touch system. Miss Standering was very patient with me. . . . For the first time since my operation I felt once more a part of the sighted community. (Krents, 1972, p. 97)

Sometimes, a reluctance to pursue professional resources and services can be traced to the mistaken notion that special education and rehabilitation services are a form of welfare or charity. That deep-rooted assumption of Western culture that demands that individuals solve their own problems and demonstrate self-sufficiency can unnecessarily prolong the adjusting process.

> In other quarters I was indeed actively discouraged from getting in touch with any of the organisations which exist in Melbourne, on the grounds, to put it bluntly, that I was not in need of charity. . . . In my case I did not want charity, but I did badly want advice. . . . I had to wrestle with my difficulties alone, and I wouldn't wish my worse enemy to go through those first months of facing blindness. (Mitchell, 1964, p. 111)

The principle of timely and appropriate resources and services applies equally to the members of the support network.

> Some people are scornful or cynical about "the experts." We are not. They are among our precious resources. Here, too, we have been fortunate, for our experts have been warm human beings, infinitely helpful. (Ulrich, 1972, p. 93)

Models

The availability of other blind individuals in the community to serve as role models is another factor influencing the adjusting process. Because of the low prevalence of blindness, many blind persons feel they are alone and unique in their adjusting struggles. Role models not only provide camaraderie but also provide an opportunity for exchange of ideas and feelings, for challenging attitudes and beliefs, for problem solving and behavior patterning. The role model can be a peer or someone much older, he can be a lay person or a professional, he can be live or in print.

> Then, too, I suppose, the students felt a sense of community with Mr. C., because he was one of the few blind members of the faculty, and the only one who was a graduate of the school. He was a model for all the students and was good, extremely good, in mobility, which automatically rated him high in the minds of the blind students. Furthermore, he was one of the few graduates since the founding of the school to go through college, and even get his M.A. (Mehta, 1957, p. 292)

While a strong, positive model may enhance the adjusting process, encounters with poor models may be detrimental to the resolution of the identity crisis, to self-acceptance and self-esteem.

> I went once or twice to the local agency for the blind, a poverty-stricken agency and a very depressing, miserable place. It was really a place to entertain the blind during the day and keep them out of harm's way. The blind shuffled in and shuffled out. They had no future. There were no jobs for the blind. They were all on welfare.... All the people who mattered to me were sighted people. (Sperber, 1976, pp. 71-72)

Employment

The degree to which a blind individual has attained or regained a status equal to his peers with comparable abilities is the degree to which he is likely to achieve self-acceptance and self-esteem. "Extended vocational inactivity may deepen and prolong depressive reactions, thus contributing to the sense of worthlessness and futility" experienced by many blind persons (Rusalem, 1972, p. 22).

> Without a job, I was nothing. . . .
> In seemingly hopeless situations such as this, I resented my blindness deeply. It made me want to strike out at the world that caused it, to get even with it. So again I became very bitter within. (Sheppard, 1956, pp. 74-75)

There is no doubt that employment is an avenue to financial independence. Through financial independence, one gains an improved sense of competence and sense of adequacy.

> I walked out of the room with a spring in my step, buoyed up by my unexpected change of fortune. The financial independence I had despaired of ever finding was mine. I felt like the condemned man who receives a reprieve just before he walks through the little green door. (Ohnstad, 1942, p. 252)

Visually impaired persons who are underemployed, who accept employment at skill levels below their abilities and training, find themselves in a serious dilemma. They desire the financial independence that comes with employment.

However, their self-esteem and self-acceptance may suffer as a result of the underemployment.

> This job gave me my first taste of financial independence, and, with it, I was getting out much more. But it was a totally dead end activity. . . . The job took away much of my disheartening boredom and desperation, but I knew that once the first excitement was over I would not be happy here indefinitely, and the search for the right job had to go on. (Edwards, 1962, p. 31)

For the recently blinded adult, the time delay before returning to work may be prolonged to provide time for the acquisition of the necessary adaptive behavior and coping skills. In some instances, the individual will require retraining for a new vocation. In other instances, the new adaptive behaviors and coping skills are sufficient to return to the previous occupation. Chevigny, soon after losing his vision, doubted that he could return to his writing profession until his colleagues, who offered to underwrite him for a year, convinced him to accept the challenge.

> As I lay in the hospital, thinking over my future and wondering what it would bring, I knew it [the presumed tragedy of blindness] was going to be the most formidable obstacle to resuming my professional life as I had known it. . . .
> With this virtual mandate, this vote of confidence from men who not only had known me for years but who—the fact was important to me at the time— are among the ablest writers in radio, I felt I had no choice but to try it. If they were willing to bet on me—well, it was up to me to take the long chance too. (Chevigny, 1946, pp. 131-135)

DEGREE OF INDEPENDENCE AND LEVEL OF SELF-ESTEEM

The meaning of independence to both the blind person and his significant others provides one of the most critical factors influencing the adjusting process. In many cultures, independence and self-sufficiency tend to be used as measures of maturity and worth. Cholden observed that "one of the clearest social attitudes toward the dependent state is that of personal devaluation. This will be felt as a lowering of self-esteem, for the receiving person is often less valued and less acceptable as a human being" (p. 100). Because of the nature of blindness, the blind person's areas of dependency are more visible than the dependency needs of others, making him more vulnerable to the effects of these negative attitudes.

> The full realization of my future dependence on people now descended on me. . . . Now, suddenly realizing that my independence would always be qualified, freedom seemed to me that most infinitely precious thing on earth. All the other drawbacks I had foreseen in the state of blindness dwindled in importance and stood only in a perspective relation to the loss of this personal freedom. (Chevigny, 1946, p. 22)

When adjusting to the many traumas of blindness, a person's emotional reactions and conflicts often fixate on the dependency aspects. The preexisting or latent chronic dependency need is the personality trait most commonly exacerbated by blindness (Blank, 1957). Perceived dependence is both a threat to the self and a temptation to succumb to the prevailing expectations (Giarratana-Oehler, 1976).

> Salvation for one who loses sight consists of avoidance of a vicious circle in which the world's fixed notion of the helplessness of the blind creates that helplessness, and their consequent exhibition of helplessness confirms the world in its fixed notion. (Chevigny, 1946, p. 88)

With society's prevailing attitudes regarding the helpless and dependent state of blind persons (see Chapter 3), many family members and friends, without thinking, cater to and thus perpetuate the perceived dependency needs of blind individuals. Naturally, the dependency needs of the young or the recently blind are more pronounced until their adaptive behaviors and coping skills are established.

> But there came a day when I sat down and did some heavy thinking. I realized that my dependence on my friends was utter and complete. I acknowledge that they were charming and behaved as though it were a pleasure to do things for me. But common sense was at work and I faced facts. . . .
> To break its [blindness] bonds, to leave the safety of my home without being in the care of a solicitous friend was a momentous decision. . . . The first time that I went out in a taxi alone was a great adventure—the greatest adventure of my blind years. . . .

Every escapade carried through successfully adds to my courage and
my sense of freedom. (Bretz, 1940, pp. 91-101)

Catering to the dependency needs after the blind individual has established his coping skills is not only unnecessary but detrimental. Parents, spouses, friends, and other
members of the support network have a tendency to overprotect and overassist.

Overprotection and overassistance are issues that arise repeat-
edly in the literature on visually impaired children. The parents
may overprotect and overassist their children because they are
concerned for the child's safety, feel guilty and consequently want
to compensate for the disability, obtain satisfaction from having
someone dependent on them, or simply are impatient with the
time it takes the child to complete the task himself. (Cook-
Clampert, 1981, p. 237)

These explanations offered for the behavior of parents are
equally applicable to explain the overprotecting and over-
assisting behaviors of other members of the support network.
Roberts (1973), analyzing the social interactions with seeing
persons from a transactional analysis perspective, observed that "an overwhelming number of the transactions are
between the parent ego state of the sighted person and the
child ego state of the blind person" (p. 58).

As a general rule, dependence is to be avoided, and
independence is to be pursued. A dependent person relies on
others for approval, is insecure and uncertain, lacks confidence in his own decisions, seeks help and constant companionship, and craves the attention and recognition of
others. On the other hand, an independent person is self-
directed and self-sufficient, is detached from the influence of
others, is free to choose his own course of action, demonstrates initiative, persistence, and curiosity, is able to solve
his problems by himself, tends to be assertive and even
aggressive, and may be more socially isolated (Coopersmith,
1967; Hamachek, 1971).

Now it's important that you understand that there were three things
I never wanted to own when I was a kid: a dog, a cane, and a guitar. In
my brain, they each meant blindness and helplessness. (Seems like

every blind blues singer I'd heard about was playing the guitar.)
It wasn't that I wanted to fool myself. Hell, I knew I was blind as a bat. But I didn't want to go limping around like I was half-dead. I didn't want to have to depend upon anyone or anything other than myself. So I learned certain tricks going around St. Augustine. And I still use 'em today. (Charles and Ritz, 1978, pp. 53-54)

In his study of preadolescent sighted boys, Coopersmith (1967) found a curvilinear relationship between level of self-esteem and degree of dependency. The high and the low self-esteem groups were certain of their status and required little confirming feedback. Boys in the medium self-esteem group were more uncertain of themselves and therefore tended to rely on others for acceptance and approval. Coopersmith suggested that dependency behaviors were associated with insecurity or deprivations in the home, indulgent or inconsistent parenting. "Dependency behaviors represent an attempt to confirm or establish a definition of one's worth or capacities" (p. 221).

There is some evidence to support the contention that, in contrast to sighted children, blind children experience even more insecurities, deprivations, indulgences, and inconsistencies, making them more vulnerable to dependency behaviors. Using the Bailer-Cromwell Children's Locus of Control Scale, Land and Vineberg (1965) studied the extent to which blind children perceived themselves as being in control of events within their environment (internal control). Comparing three matched groups of eighteen children each (residential school blind children, public school blind children, and sighted children) they found that both blind groups scored significantly lower for internal control than the sighted, that the amount of vision of the blind subjects was not correlated with locus of control, and that age was positively correlated with internal locus of control. In another study, Gomulcki (1961) suggested that blind children's higher achievement in some subject areas may be associated with parents who encouraged independent or self-reliant behaviors in their children.

Chapman (1978) described the acquisition of independence as a gradual process. The blind child "cannot make the transition from childhood to adolescence in one step, and needs the chance increasingly to make his own decisions, decide for himself what to eat, what to wear, what do do, what new pursuits to follow and what new responsibilities to undertake" (p. 118). She stated that the overly dependent blind adolescent "may have had insufficient opportunities for independence, even at the level of making decisions about small matters. . . . Conversely inappropriate reactions of belligerence can be evident if he has had to struggle with adults for the chance to express his personality in his own way" (p.118).

Everyone finds himself at some point on the independent-dependent continuum. Many blind persons tend to polarize at one extreme or the other. The unrealistically dependent blind person seeks emotional and physical security in the total care demanded. The unrealistically independent blind person tends to find himself attempting dangerous and foolish tasks, or places himself and others in awkward and embarrassing situations.

> When we finished eating, he gave me the money to pay the check. "I've got a friend in Waterloo who insists on paying the bills himself," he remarked. "He has his wife lead him up to the counter, and he gropes around looking for the place to put the money. She could just as well pay the bill and it would be better for everybody. He claims he doesn't feel like a man if he doesn't do those things. I think that's silly. If you can do things as well as a sighted person, do them. If not, where unimportant things like this are concerned, let them. That's the way I feel." (Moore, 1960, p. 26)

According to Lowenfeld (1975), visually handicapped persons responding to the dependency aspects of blindness tend to react either with hostility and aggression, with submissiveness and compliance, or with a more balanced willingness to accept needed assistance when the circumstances of a given situation seem to warrant the help. "The last of the three alternatives demands considerable ego strength and a self-concept that is positive enough to induce resistance to dependency" (p. 265).

Coburn (1964) put the problem of dependency into proper

perspective when he observed that "without dependency, rugged individualism becomes ruthless individualism.... Dependency is not something bad, but something good, ... not something unusual, but something normal" (p. 37). After observing that one can have too much or too little of a good thing, he continued "the extremely independent person is usually a sick and unhappy person. . . . Man is not an independent animal" (pp. 37-38). According to Coburn, the root of the problem is the erroneous overglorification of independence and the condemnation of normal dependence by society. The suddenly blinded may feel inferior because he can no longer maintain society's false standard of independence and may feel he is no longer capable of self-sufficiency or self-respect.

Fitts (1970) compared the normal self to a wheel with two equal halves: the "offering self" and the "seeking self." The spokes that intersected both halves of the wheel were labeled Involvement, Responsibility, Freedom, Empathetic Understanding, Openness, Caring, and Acceptance. The hub and the rim, he said, defined the inner and outer limits of these qualities, while the tire represented firm but flexible consistency.

Fitts's wheel illustrates the healthy balance between the giving self and the receiving self, between independence and dependence. The wheel becomes out-of-round or flattened on one side when either the "offering self" or the "seeking self" diminishes. Referring to two unbalanced wheels, one with a diminished "offering self" and the other with a diminished "seeking self," Fitts commented "the only way these two wheels could work very well together would be if they were placed side by side and fastened together to constitute one wheel," for example, a "kind of symbiotic relationship that exists in some unhealthy mother-child relationships" (p. 36).

An analysis of the "offering self" of others and the "seeking self" of VI provides some insights into the dynamics of the relationship between perceived dependency and VI's self-esteem. The manner in which assistance is offered by others impacts directly on VI's sense of value and worth. The manner in which assistance is received by VI reveals something of his own self-esteem needs. When VI learns to understand the various motives and drives of the "offering self" of others and when he learns to understand his own feelings and reactions, he is then in a better position to minimize the negative effect on his own self-esteem.

Assistance Offered by Others

There are many possible ways of categorizing assistance offered. Welsh (1980) described three types of assistance offered as "those which are unsolicited and unnecessary, those which are unsolicited and necessary, and those which are solicited" (p. 255). Rather than categorizing types of assistance, the following analysis attempts to describe types of responses people exhibit when they offer assistance. The labels are for discussion purposes only. Although the sighted person will tend to react predominately in one of the ways described, he may employ many of the other types, depending on the circumstances and the mood of the moment. Hopefully, the quality of his responses will improve and he will become more comfortable with the role of offering assistance as he becomes better acquainted with the visually impaired person.

The underlying motivations for offering assistance are varied and numerous. Some demonstrate a genuine care and concern by promoting in the other "growth, development, maturity, improved functioning, improved coping with life" (Rogers, 1961, pp. 39-40). There are those with a lack of knowledge and experience in such matters who approach the situation simply out of curiosity. Some offer assistance as a matter of routine course because it is expected of them. Still others are motivated by pity. "Pity for another implies inferiority. . . . There may be inner need to place others in an inferior position, and pity is a perfect excuse, for it cloaks its purpose in what seems the highest of social sanctions. . . . In all these individuals, the rejection of their pity causes anger to break through" (Chevigny and

Braverman, 1950, pp. 150-152). Regardless of the motivation, many approach the helping task with fear and anxiety simply because they are unsure of the best or appropriate way.

The following types emerge from an analysis of those who are in a position to offer assistance.

1. The Fearful Avoider: There are individuals who, upon observing a blind person in apparent need of help, are so anxious and fearful that they avoid any contact with the blind person. The fearful avoider may walk across the street or use another door to avoid "an unpleasant encounter."

> One, with unusual candor and an actor's lack of embarrassment, said, "I couldn't go to see you when you were in the hospital because I was afraid that if what happened to you should happen to me I wouldn't be able to take it—and I couldn't think of anything to say to you that I would mean in all honesty." (Chevigny, 1946, p. 198)

2. The Forceful Dominator: Presuming to know the extent and type of help needed, the dominator proceeds forcefully to impose his brand of assistance. He does not consult the blind person nor does he take suggestions. The dominator must be in control at all times.

> I can never forget my distress at the ladies' luncheon when the fellow-guest at my right "managed" everything for me. Her desire to help me was touching but I became utterly fatigued with trying to dodge the unpredictable, unannounced movements of her hands about my plate as she reached across to get my soup spoon and put it into the soup, "all nice and ready for you," and later to get the fork and arrange it "real handy" on my plate. Since I was accustomed to doing all these things for myself, I grew more and more confused. The final torment came with the dessert, which was sliced fresh peaches. Over my protest as well as over the peaches, she poured a lavish amount of cream and then, scooping up a spoonful at a time, she passed the spoon to me, admonishing me to "Chew it well." At the end I fully expected her to say, "Now, let me wipe your little mouth and take off your bib." (McCoy, 1963, p. 107)

3. The Condescending Patronizer: This individual sees himself as a precious gift especially to the "unfortunate blind." The view that the blind person is inferior is

revealed in the condescending manner the patronizer uses when talking down to the blind person.

Of all the attitudes which seeing people can display to the blind, the most infuriating is the habit some have of taking it easy when they are playing chess or any other game with a blind person. . . . When I am playing an opponent for the first time, I have noticed, too often to put it down to coincidence, that he just happens to make an irreparable mistake a move or two after I have thrown away my queen. Before he took my queen he has strenuously urged me to take the move back, but he will not consider making another move instead of his disastrous one. (Edwards, 1962, pp. 39-40)

4. **The Reluctant Inquirer:** After observing a definite need, this individual is reluctant to discuss the problem for fear of offending or hurting the blind person's feelings. The approach is a cautious inquiry as to the blind person's level of awareness of the potential problem. If desired or needed, the problem is explained, but the blind person is permitted to assume the decision-making role.

I remember meeting a friend in the street some years ago. She had always been fond of clothes and took great pleasure in her appearance. Now she was old and had lost her sight, but she was fiercely independent, and, while still living alone, struggled to keep her standards. She had on odd stockings, noticeably odd. I thought she was going to the local shop and had no intention of commenting, but she had no basket, and she wore a hat and carried a handbag and gloves, and I decided something more was afoot. With some hesitation I told her. She clutched me by the arm and more or less commanded in the nicest way, that I should go back and help her find a pair of stockings. I did this and she confided that she was going to a very special party and was being picked up at the bus stop by her host. She was so grateful for this small service, which I had almost thought of as interference. (Lunt, 1965, pp. 106-107)

5. **The Helpful Inquirer:** Making no assumptions about the blind person's need for assistance, the helpful inquirer makes verbal contact with the blind person and courteously asks if there is any way he may be of assistance. In other words, the helpful inquirer simply makes himself available if and when assistance is needed. This approach leaves the blind person in control of the situation. A school administrator exhibited the atti-

tudes of a helpful inquirer in his conversation with Krents.

"Whatever the problem, I stand ready to alleviate it in any way I can. In short, all that I'm trying to say is that you are not alone, that there is someone who is behind you all the way who would like to help whenever you feel that help is necessary." (Krents, 1972, p. 239)

6. **The Obligated Significant Other:** There are individuals who offer assistance because they feel morally obligated to do so. The parent, sibling, or spouse finds himself bound by a relationship in which he has very little choice.

I didn't ask Mary Sue [a younger sister] to lead Davey around very often. We have always tried very hard not to expect her to stop her playing to help him, but occasionally we did ask her. Just as any parent asks a child for help, for assistance. And usually she did it graciously, towing him along like a small sturdy tugboat. But sometimes she stuck out her lip and glared at me when I asked her. Then she would think better of it and take Davey's hand. (Henderson, 1954, p. 174)

7. **The Available Friend:** A friendship is a give and take relationship. A friend willingly offers assistance but, at a later time, will seek assistance from the blind person. The relationship is mutually beneficial, rewarding, and satisfying. Each assumes the decision-making role when it is appropriate. Hocken's relationship with Anita was that of a friend, mutually satisfying.

There was one thing I could not manage on my own, and for which I had to rely a great deal on Anita. That was dress sense. It is very difficult to pick the right clothes if you can't see the color and can only touch the garments to get an idea of the material and style. When I went into a shop in the days before I lived with Anita, it was very often a case of Never-mind-the-quality, feel-the-width. But with her advice I could wear clothes that I knew were fashionable. (Hocken, 1977, p. 82)

Assistance Received by VI

When assistance is offered by others, VI may respond with any one of a number of possible reactions. Although they tend to fall predominantly into one of the following categories, he may occasionally employ any of the others depending on the circumstances and his mood.

As was mentioned above, others offering assistance may be uncertain and anxious about the approach or method. This uncertainty or anxiety may be erroneously interpreted by VI as pity or condescension. At the same time, VI may be uncertain or anxious about obtaining needed assistance. VI's uncertainty and anxiety may be interpreted by others as further proof of incompetence or helplessness.

Assistance that is unclear or ambiguous, that is offered without explanation, only serves to confuse and bewilder VI. There is nothing more disconcerting than for VI to hear someone holler "watch out!" In the first place, VI may not know whether he is being addressed. Second, he doesn't know how to interpret the attempted assistance—should he withdraw, stand still, jump, or run.

> When I crossed intersections . . . and was carefully working my way through the heavy traffic, someone from the sidewalk would shout, "Watch out!" as though it were only a matter of seconds before a car would run me over. I used to get paralyzed with fear and lose all sense of direction and control. . . . No sooner was "Watch out" bellowed than I would lose my nerve. (Mehta, 1957, p. 262)

The following types emerge from an analysis of those who are in the position to accept assistance.

1. The Super-independent Refuser: There are some blind individuals who are unrealistically independent, refusing any and all offers of assistance. They seem to have a need to prove to the world that they can be independent and self-sufficient.

> Maurice said . . . "Believe me, though, time will . . ."
>
> "Leave me alone with your blasted time!" Robert cried angrily, jumping up. "Everyone prates about healing time. . . . I've been blind for three years, and for every moment of those three years I've cursed my fate."
>
> He wanted to run from the room but ran into a table and overturned it. I took his arm to help him. "Leave me alone," he cried. "I don't need any help!" He took another step and stumbled over a chair. His face was distorted, his hands shook. Maurice rose from his chair and, as if he saw where he was going, went up to him. He took Robert's arm and led him from the room. (Vajda, 1974, p. 48)

2. The Self-conscious Retreater: Having a goal or objective in mind, the retreater senses that assistance is needed but is too self-conscious or embarrassed to "impose" on someone else. For example, the blind high schooler who desires to attend the homecoming football festivities decides to stay at home rather than ask someone for a ride. The habitual retreater experiences many unfulfilled goals and objectives.

3. The Wishful Waiter: When needing assistance, VI stands around passively hoping against hope that someone will come along to offer assistance. Naturally, it is incumbent upon the waiter to assume as helpless a pose as possible in order to motivate another to approach him.

> I used up an immense amount of time simply getting from my dorm to class. There would usually be someone around to help, but too often those who came to my assistance did so grudgingly, declaring that they were late for class themselves. (Sullivan and Gill, 1975, p. 108)

4. The Realistic Seeker: The seeker knows the nature and extent of the assistance required, assertively seeks this assistance, and graciously refuses all other. The confident seeker is usually in control, able to manage most situations effectively. In addition, this person seeks opportunities to give as well as receive.

> I had faced the fact squarely that I would have to live with my blindness. Then I tried to decide how best I could manage, without leaning too much on others, and yet being willing to accept help when I really needed it. . . .
> I would have to be honest about admitting my limitations, and willing to tell my friends when I needed their aid. (Dahl, 1962, pp. 131-132)

5. The Reluctant Acceptor: Sometimes VI is put in an awkward position. He does not need the assistance being thrust upon him but to avoid an argument, to avoid further embarrassment or to avoid offending someone, VI reluctantly accepts the offered assistance.

> When some people notice a blind man, they seem to feel they must do something positive for him, or at least give him something. Travelling

on a tram in Melbourne one day before I started smoking, a woman about to get off stopped next to me, thrust a packet of cigarettes into my hand and insisted that I took them.

As in the case of an offer of a seat I do not need, it seems simpler in the long run to comply. Provided no big amount is involved, to refuse gifts is not worth the embarrassment to all concerned. But I loathe being placed in these situations. Wanting to be as independent as I can, I find it ridiculous to realize that I am regarded this way, to be taken as someone needing and expecting gifts and special treatment. (Edwards, 1962, p. 171)

6. **The Passive Acceptor:** This individual accepts all assistance offered whether he needs it or not. He has not learned how to graciously refuse unneeded help and so finds himself passively accepting all help. In its extreme form, passive acceptance may become a life-style of dependency.

If through lack of use you let your mind and faculties rot, if you let yourself drift into a state of parasitic dependence on the life around you, the decay in you may spread and affect others. Parasitism, only taking from life and not giving to it, is terribly dangerous, and I would say that it is harder not to become a parasite if you are blind than if you are afflicted with almost any other disability. (Mitchell, 1964, p. 14)

7. **The Habitual Demander:** When help is constantly available whether it is needed or not, VI may come to expect it or even demand it. Unless taught otherwise, VI may come to view assistance as "a right of blindness." This unhealthy demanding attitude is frequently unsciously learned from the good intentions of others who indiscriminantly cater to the needs, wants, and desires of VI.

The dynamics of the interaction between VI's "seeking self" and the "offering self" of others will vary from one situation to the next. If a "Forceful Dominator" encounters a "Superindependent Refuser," hostilities may surface quickly. Resentments tend to build when the "Obligated Significant Other" attempts to passify the "Habitual Demander." When the "Condescending Patronizer" meets the "Wishful Waiter," the needs of both may be met but at a cost to VI's self-esteem.

If the relationship between VI and others is to be more than simply a casual acquaintance, then opportunities for mutual give and take must be sought and acted upon. There is a loss of self-esteem and self-respect when VI perceives himself always in the receiving mode. Extending oneself toward others requires initiative and ingenuity involving a certain amount of personal risk. Even at a time when Backhall was experiencing his own trauma of the onset of blindness, he was able to reach out to another.

> He [a patient in the hospital, at the time the author had lost his sight following four operations] explained, "I was feeling so utterly depressed, I felt I must talk to someone. Nurse told me to go and see Mr. Blackhall. He'd cheer me up."
>
> It transpired that he had had a cyst removed from his eyelid, a comparatively simple operation. The loneliness was weighing heavily upon him and he came to me to cheer him up!.
>
> I hardly deserved such a reputation at that moment, but I thought it was quite the nicest thing which could be said about me. When we are able to help someone else, it does not take anything away from us. It adds to our own strength. There was I, at the lowest possible ebb, and there was he, a little lonely. . . .
>
> I never sank quite so low again after this experience. (Blackhall, 1962, p. 111)

> *If* we are willing to risk some Involvement with others and *if* we offer *democratic* Involvement, characterized by Responsibility and Freedom, and *if* we concentrate upon complete, two-way communication (Understanding and Openness), *then* we will also be able to offer Caring and Acceptance to others. If then we seek from others what we offer *to* them, we will usually get what we seek and all parties will move toward greater self-actualization and a better world. (Fitts, 1970, p. 38)

SUMMARY

This chapter has identified some of the factors that impact either positively or negatively on the adjusting process. VI brings a set of characteristics with him into the adjusting process that become important determiners. Some of these variables include personality, coping experiences, prior attitudes toward blindness, intelligence, age, degree and stability of vision, additional complications, and philosophical beliefs. Other important determiners are defined by factors external to VI, such as the role of the ophthalmologist, personal support network, professional resources and services, models, and employment. Since perceived dependence is one of the most critical factors in the adjusting process, the role of assistance offered by others and assistance received by VI was examined and analyzed in terms of the potential impact on VI's self-esteem. Learning to make the most of these variables provides the maximum opportunity for VI's self-esteem to flourish.

Section IV
FOSTERING SELF-ESTEEM

Chapter 10

GUIDELINES AND SUGGESTED ACTIVITIES

"**A** good self concept is passed to children through demonstrating more hope than fear, more trust than distrust, more integrity than deceit" (Rapp, 1974, p. 14). The same principle is true for developing and maintaining a good self-concept in persons of any age. Adults, too, need to experience hope, trust, and integrity.

Because of the reflected appraisals discussed in Chapter 4 and the expectations discussed in Chapter 5, frequently academic or vocational achievements become measures of a successful program. In reality, they may be very unreliable indicators. "If a client completes a training program, or is placed in a job, but still views *himself* as worthless, inadequate or undesirable, he may not be truly rehabilitated even though his records are closed and he is reported as a 'success' case" (Fitts, 1972, p. 9). In other words, the level of self-acceptance and self-esteem may be better indicators of a successful program.

Special education and rehabilitation workers have given far too little recognition and attention to the critical role that self-concept or, more specifically, self-esteem plays in the habilitation or rehabilitation process (Delafield, 1976). Lowenfeld (1975) observed "I have always contended that the self-assertive and even slightly aggressive blind person has a better chance to find employment than the one who is submissive or meek" (p. 144). He continued by expressing the conviction that unfortunately most professionals tend to expect if not demand passive and compliant behavior, when they should be encouraging a more independent life-style. "Cultivation of self-assertiveness based on a positive self-concept appears to be an important task of schools and agencies for the blind" (p. 145).

Whether professionals or lay people like it or not, they are active participants in the shaping and molding of the self-esteem of the people with whom they associate. Furthermore, the changes they effect may be either positive or negative (Canfield and Wells, 1976). To effect a positive change is not easy; it requires time, patience, and many positive experiences. "The self-concept cannot be changed by words alone or by intellectual knowledge. For better or for worse, the self-concept is changed only by experience" (LaBenne and Greene, 1969, p. 121).

Consistant, persistent, and credible positive messages from trusted significant others facilitate a positive change in self-esteem. It requires a concerted team effort of lay people (parents, other family members, and friends) and professionals (teachers, rehabilitation counselors, nurses, and social workers) who are experienced in working with blind persons. The professional may need to provide some leadership for this team effort.

GUIDELINES FOR WORKING WITH BLIND PERSONS

Many lay people as well as professionals have never encountered a blind person and therefore experience considerable apprehension and anxiety about their role. The following guidelines (Blechman, 1970) and suggestions are offered, particularly in light of the first three sections of this book.

1. Blind people are, first, people with the same basic needs of love, acceptance, and feelings of worth as everyone else.
2. Perceiving a world without vision is a very real and valid experience. The nonvisual interpretation of the social and physical environment must be accepted and

respected without unnecessarily imposing a visual frame of reference.

"I hear something," he said, "Listen, Mummy."

"I don't hear anything," I said, too sleepy from the wind and sun to even listen. "It's just the ocean."

"No, no, it's something else, something high and shrill. Listen."

Al [his father] opened his eyes. "It's a sea gull," he said, pointing it out to me.

Davey hugged his knees tightly against his chest, "I heard it," he boasted. "I heard it first. A sea gull. Oh, boy!"

And it did not matter to him that he could not see the gull, silver and white, curving through the air like a polished thing in the sun, for he had heard it first. (Henderson, 1954, p. 194)

3. Emphasis should be placed on the positive, the "I can's," the abilities, and the assets while at the same time maintaining a realistic perspective regarding any possible problems or limitations.

4. Instructions must be articulated clearly, without relying on facial expressions and body language to convey meaning. Occasionally it may be necessary, with the blind person's permission, to manipulate his body or body parts to demonstrate the desired motion. The following excerpt illustrates the need for carefully thought-out instruction and the need to anticipate the desired response.

"Tell me when I turn it on and when I turn it off," Jim would ask. I told him, even though I saw no light.

After a few days, he realized that I was basing my answers on the heat I felt when the flashlight was on. I hadn't been trying to kid him: I'd merely told him when the light was on or off, as he had asked. Maybe I should have told him I couldn't see a doggone thing, but that was something I didn't want to believe, much less say. It was simply a matter of fact that I could tell when the light was on and when it wasn't, in my own way. (Boswell, 1969, p. 61)

5. Visually impaired persons must be encouraged to accomplish tasks independently, with intervention only when necessary. Occasionally this will require extra time, especially when newly acquired skills are being employed.

6. Visually impaired persons like everyone else need the encouragment provided by praise for genuine accomplishments and tasks well done. However, false praise for achievements that are ordinary or routine can be detrimental.

7. Significant others need to formulate and carefully maintain realistic expectations that are commensurate with the blind person's abilities and skills. Blindness should never be used as an excuse for unacceptable behavior. The same behavioral standards should be applied to the blind and sighted alike.

8. Visually impaired persons must learn to set realistic aspirations based on a thorough understanding of interests and desires, strengths and limitations, abilities and inabilities, acquired and potential skills, viewing all these traits and characteristics in the broadest sense and not just as they relate to blindness.

9. Visually impaired persons rely on candid and honest feedback from others to determine the social acceptability of their appearance and behaviors.

> As well as helping with my clothes, Anita was also able to tell me if my hair looked right. She was my mirror. But the best thing about her was that she treated me as a paid-up member of the human race. She had a great sense of honesty and never made embarrassing allowances for the fact that I could not see. (Hocken, 1977, p. 82)

10. Questions about vision, sex, careers, relationships, etc. require frank and accurate responses. When the information requested is not known, a simple acknowledgement of that fact and an expression of a willingness to find someone who does have the desired information would be helpful.

11. Conversations with visually impaired persons should be natural. There is no need for shouting and no need to avoid visually oriented words such as "look" and "see," as they are also part of a blind person's vocabulary.

12. When a sighted person is approaching a visually impaired person and it is not immediately apparent what, if any, help is desired, the blind person should simply be

asked. Frequently problems can be solved with the application of a little common sense, and usually the simplest approach is the best.

13. Active involvement in the community social, recreational, and civic affairs facilitates fuller assimilation. Personal and social competence is more important than anything else to achieve better integration into the community.

14. Anyone working with the visually impaired must become aware of his own feelings and attitudes toward blindness and resolve any problems before inadvertently communicating negative or derogatory attitudes.

These guidelines and suggestions are but a few of the techniques and approaches that are useful when working with persons who are blind. They are concerned more with methodologies that are particularly unique to the blind than with general principles and guidelines that foster self-acceptance and self-esteem in others. To learn more of the specific adaptive coping skills and the use of specialized aids and devices, it would be necessary to receive further training in special education or rehabilitation of the visually handicapped. These techniques and devices are designed to assist the blind person to cope successfully with the problems mentioned in Chapter 2: personal and home management, travel, reading and writing, recreation, and employment. In addition to the unique methodologies of working with a blind person, there are even more basic principles and guidelines that govern the development of self-acceptance and self-esteem.

One of the disabling myths, according to DeLoach (1981) is "the omniscience of the experts" (p. 43). Professionals and lay persons alike can assist the blind person toward self-acceptance and self-esteem. They must bear in mind the goals of the adjusting process: acceptance of one's disability, a healthy self-acceptance and self-esteem, assimilation into society, and adequate social techniques and psychological mechanisms to cope with the behavior of others (DeLoach, 1981). The professional or lay person must be a motivator who can encourage the visually handicapped person toward his potential. Good education and rehabilitation programs should focus their efforts on helping blind persons move toward optimum self-sufficiency, self-fulfillment, and self-actualization (Fitts, 1972). It will require both empathetic understanding and firm resolve to assist blind persons toward these goals.

> Since my loss of normal vision I have a strange inner paradox as I counsel people. I am enormously empathetic when people speak to me of their hurts, losses, and surprises. I know the feeling: I have been there, I know it hurts. I know the panic, the despair, the awful struggle to reach for help and healing, and my hands go out quickly to those who experience these things. But I am also impatient with the snifflers, complainers, those who think they cannot or will not try to cope with their altered situations. The combination makes me gentle but tough. (Kemper, 1977, p. 113)

ATTITUDES AND BEHAVIORS THAT FOSTER AFFECTIVE GROWTH

> I was helped most by those who had themselves walked my path.... I was helped by those who did not feel sorry for me.... I was helped by those who had something to do and did it.... I was helped by those who listened to me when I wanted to talk.... I was helped by those with a sense of humor.... I was helped by those who were loyal. (Kemper, 1977, p. 128)

The sensitive, concerned lay person as well as the professional working with blind persons can exert a powerful influence on the adjusting process toward self-acceptance and self-esteem. Since there is no unique psychology of the blind, the attributes and behaviors that maximize self-acceptance and self-esteem in visually impaired persons are the same as the attributes and behaviors that maximize self-acceptance and self-esteem in all persons. A review of Sections II and III and pertinent literature (Canfield and Wells, 1976; Dobson, 1974; LaBenne and Greene, 1969; McCandless, 1977) suggests that the following characteristics seem to be associated with fostering affective growth in others.

Characteristic Attributes

1. He is self-accepting, with a healthy self-esteem.
2. He is positive toward others, actively seeking the value and worth in others.
3. He is not skeptical, cynical, or unduly suspicious of others.
4. He is accepting of others, their contributions and efforts, their talents and faults, their strengths and weaknesses.
5. He is genuinely and personally interested in each individual, taking time to listen to each.
6. He is able to see things from other people's perspectives, thus increasing his capacity for empathy.
7. He possesses good interpersonal skills and is able to resolve conflicts that may arise.
8. He is able to receive as well as give in personal relationships and is able to teach others to do the same.
9. He is supportive of others.

Characteristic Behaviors

1. He develops and maintains strong interpersonal relationships with a variety of individuals.
2. He structures experiences so that others can "discover" ideas and relationships for themselves rather than authoritatively imposing his own ideas and views on others.
3. He sets expectations of others that are in harmony with their talents and abilities.
4. He designs activities for others that insure maximum opportunity for success.
5. He does not view other's inability to meet his expectations as "a failure" but rather views it as a positive learning experience for both.
6. He tends to employ criterion referenced measures, thus using the individual as his own standard, rather than employing norm-referenced measures that force comparison and competition with others.
7. He avoids correcting others in public and refrains from

using sarcasm in that correction.
8. He actively seeks the ideas and opinions of others.

Characteristic Assisting Behaviors

1. He assists others to develop good interpersonal skills and relationships.
2. He assists others to understand themselves better, to clarify their perceptions of their personal attributes in a wholesome and accepting atmosphere.
3. He enables others to present themselves positively, to capitalize on their strengths and inner resources.
4. He assists others by encouraging them with a positive "you can do it" attitude.
5. He assists others to set realistic aspirations that sometimes means saying "let's try" to an unrealistic aspiration.
6. He facilitates independence, others doing for themselves, rather than his doing things to or for them.
7. He provides the support necessary to enable others to recognize and think through their own problems, to search for alternative solutions and to choose a course of action.
8. He stimulates others to mobilize effectively available resources and services.
9. He encourages others to establish and utilize relevant standards and values for measuring their own performances rather than relying on external evaluations.

Anyone dedicated to building self-acceptance and self-esteem in others will find that it is not an easy task. He must first establish himself as trustworthy and credible so that the message he shares will also be accepted. Effecting a positive change in a person's self-concept requires consistency, persistency, and repetition. The change takes place slowly over a long period of time and, in fact, may take place so slowly as to go unnoticed. Self-esteem is not a subject in the school or rehabilitation curriculum but is a by-product of the attitudes and activities of the entire team of people who interact with the visually impaired person.

Fostering affective growth is not to be confused with therapeutic counseling. The development of self-acceptance and self-esteem as described in this book is a very practical, continuous process in which everyone participates, whether they like it or not. It is the responsibility of the professional or lay person to recognize the signs of the more serious personality problems and to refer for professional counseling or psychiatric help. Some of the more serious problems described in Chapter 8 included persistent denial, extreme withdrawal, active fantasy life, deep depression, suicidal tendencies, and persistent unresolved hostility. Fortunately, these extreme maladaptive behaviors are the exception rather than the rule.

ACTIVITIES TO STIMULATE AFFECTIVE GROWTH

Although building self-esteem requires active planning and purposeful activities, it is usually most effective when it remains as a hidden agenda. The activities offered in this section can appear to be incidental to other learning objectives. For example, in a typing or braille lesson, the visually impaired person can practice his skill by brailling or typing his response to one of the activities described in this section. There may be time for an activity when waiting for the cake to bake in a cooking lesson. Some of the following suggestions may be presented simply as part of "fun and game" time. Others might be appropriate as a topic of conversation at mealtime or when riding in a car or bus. In other words, fostering affective growth can be a hidden agenda for any time and any place.

Some of the suggested activities are most effective when working individually, one on one. Others are more effective when used with a group of visually impaired persons, such as in an informal group. This should not be confused with, or construed as, a therapy group that requires a professional trained leader. Some activities can be very effective in a mixed group of both blind and sighted. Sometimes, an intimate group of family or friends is best, while other times a group of casual acquaintances or strangers is better. The choice of timing, setting, and group composition all require a sensitivity to the needs of each individual. The activities are designed to help the visually impaired person—

1. work through some of the phases of adjusting;
2. gain in self-understanding by clarifying and refining his perceptions of his personal attributes and self-concept;
3. confront and if necessary modify his own feelings and attitudes toward himself, toward blindness, and toward others;
4. disclose himself to another by sharing his likes and dislikes, aspirations and expectations, standards and values;
5. develop a concern for others, their interests and desires, their joys and frustrations, their standards and values;
6. understand and enhance relationships with others;
7. identify and discuss any concerns or problems related to blindness: cause and prognosis of visual loss, heredity issues, effective coping strategies, management of the sighted public, etc;
8. improve his self-confidence and self-esteem.

The number(s) following the activity keys that activity to the above goal(s) it is designed to accomplish. The activities are offered with the intent that they will serve to stimulate further development of other activities. They are not grouped according to goals or topics, but are arranged more or less according to the age for which they are appropriate, children first, then youth, and finally adults, though many can be used with modification for any age.

Not all of the suggested activities focus on the positive, the strengths, or the valued. Self-esteem is enhanced not only by experiences that emphasize the positive but also by involvement in situations that encourage the recognition and understanding of the negative, the limitations, and the devalued. Some of the suggestions that appear to be self-defeating from a self-esteem point of view are, in fact, promoting healthy affective growth.

Since the development of self-esteem in blind persons parallels the development of self-esteem in all persons

(Mangold, 1982), some activities in the following list have been adapted from ideas recommended for the general population (Alley, 1978; Canfield and Wells, 1976; Dinkmeyer, 1970; Dupont et al., 1974; Locke and Gerler, 1981; Palomares and Ball, 1972; Stevens, 1973).

1. Make attractive posters using the following ideas and utilize them as discussion stimulators (6, 8):
   I have to love me before I can love you.
   I need someone to love and someone who loves me.
   I'm me and I'm OK 'cause God don't make no junk.
   Decide who owns the problem.
   Free to be me.
   Think for yourself, your friends may be wrong.
   You're special ... one of a kind.
   Dare to fail.
   Your behavior will match your concept of yourself.
   To have everyone's approval means giving up the self.
   Have the courage to try.
   To use friends is to lose friends.
   Your choice of friends is your propaganda.

2. Seat everyone in a circle. The first person introduces himself by using his first name accompanied by a complimentary adjective beginning with the same letter, i.e. Considerate Connie or Dandy David. The next person repeats all previous alliterations and adds his own (2, 5).

3. Hand out slips of paper and ask the participants to list the three character traits that they most admire in others and would like best to have in themselves. Fold the papers, shuffle, and redistribute them. See how many people can be identified by the three traits they had listed (2, 5).

4. Have each member of the group list five experiences he has had that no one else in the group has had. Discuss the uniqueness of each individual (2, 4, 8).

5. Identify one member of the group and have each of the other members write down one complimentary comment about that person, without signing their names. Repeat

the procedure for each member of the group. Collect the comments and sort them by participants. Share the compiled comments privately with the one being described (2,5).

6. Ask each of the group members to identify three people who love him and make him feel good. In how many different ways do they show their love and concern? (1,6, 8).

7. Ask the students to list as many different ways as possible to solve the following problems (6, 7):
   a. You left your lunch money at home and it's time for lunch.
   b. While at a social function, you discover you have on mismatched socks.
   c. A stranger has bumped you and caused you to drop your books and papers.

8. Have the participants complete open-ended statements that focus on relationships with others and then discuss the responses (3, 4).
   People bug me when they _____.
   I helped _____.
   I feel sorry for _____.
   People who agree with me make me feel _____.

9. Discuss what could have happened to make a person feel (a) angry, (b) contented, (c) disgusted, and (d) excited (5, 6).

10. Ask each member of the group to gather objects that are of value to him and put them in a box. Ask each to share the significance of the items in his "treasure chest" (4, 8).

11. Ask the participants to describe five activities they currently enjoy doing by themselves and five others they enjoy doing with others. Ask which they have learned from others and which they have discovered for themselves. Then ask: What enjoyment have you given someone else today? (5, 6).

12. Develop several sets of cards using adjectives (personal qualities, values, etc.) in large type and braille. Have the

visually impaired person sort them into three stacks: "Most like me," "Less like me," and "Least like me." (2).

13. Have each member of the group develop and deliver a three minute speech about himself (4, 8).

14. Have the group discuss ways to contribute to the welfare of the other members in their families (5, 8).

15. Ask each member of the group to write down an annoying trait or behavior they observe in another person, followed by having them write five of the most positive characteristics of that person. Then ask them to do the same for themselves. Discuss the effects of focusing on the positive rather than the negative (2, 6).

16. Have the participants complete these open-ended statements that focus on personal attributes and then discuss the responses (2,4):
    The thing I most value is _____.
    I am best at _____.
    If I could change one thing about myself I would _____.
    I want to be _____.

17. Have each member of the group list five qualities of a good friend and five qualities of a poor friend. Discuss the extent to which the friendship is a two way street (6).

18. Role play a situation in which a visually impaired person is being teased or ridiculed about aspects of blindness (3, 7).

19. Identify people who behave in a confident manner and others who do not. Discuss the difference. Have participants portray confidence as a banquet speaker, as a cook, and as a roller skater. Then have the group members portray the same activities with a lack of confidence (8).

20. Put the names of each member of the group on a separate piece of paper. Have each member draw a name. This becomes his candidate for group president. Have each member write down as many reasons as possible in support of his candidate. Have each member share his list of qualifications to see if the group can

identify the potential candidate (5, 8).

21. Have each member select three objects: (a) the one that they are most like, (b) the one that they are least like, and (c) the one that they would like to become. For example: I am like a piano, I make music. I am least like a chair, always sat upon. I would like to be a tree, strong and tall (2).

22. Pick one member of the group to give a speech about himself while pretending that he feels worthless. Pick another to do the same while pretending to feel superior to others. Discuss how people react to both types (6).

23. Role play situations that are intended to produce feelings of (a) indifference, (b) happiness, (c) embarrassment, (d) respect, and (e) discouragement (2, 3).

24. Have each participant identify a decision he made independently and a decision that was influenced by others. Discuss the following questions (3, 8):
    a. Are you easily influenced? If so, by whom? Why?
    b. Do you influence other people's decisions? How does this make you feel?
    c. Is it wrong to rely on others for decisions?

25. Attention-getting behaviors are used by individuals of all ages. Discuss some appropriate and some inappropriate methods of capturing the attention of others. Illustrate how the classification of appropriate or inappropriate could change with age and situation. Role play some attention-getting behaviors (2, 6).

26. Ask the participants to illustrate how a situation or event can produce both good feelings and bad feelings at the same time (1, 3).

27. Have the participants plan and execute a group activity, but secretly assign one of the members to display the "I can't" attitude. Discuss people's reactions to the "I can't" attitude (1, 3).

28. Play the Ungame™ with the group (Published by the Ungame Co., P.O. Box 6382, Anaheim, Ca. 92806) (2, 4, 6, 8).

29. Discuss the fact that a put-down can make a person feel

unhappy. Ask the participants to give examples and to analyze reasons for their use (5, 6).

30. Using the descriptions of the types of relationships found in Chapter 4, have one member of the group role play the blind person. Have another member select one of the types and portray this in his encounter with the blind person, allowing the group to guess which type of relationship is being portrayed (1, 3, 7).

31. Have your group members comment on the saying "Everybody's doing it." Ask them to what extent blindness interferes with participating in what everyone else does (1, 3, 7).

32. Read some statements to which the group members must either agree, disagree, or pass. This works best when the participants have to move to a specific location in the room to indicate their choice and those either agreeing or disagreeing must give a reason for their choice. Suggested statements: "Blindness is an inconvenience," "There are many things blind people cannot do," "I like me" (1. 2, 3).

33. Discuss ways of resolving the difference of opinion in the following situations (1, 7):
    a. Your parents think you ought to get a part-time job (babysitting, selling greeting cards, etc.); you don't think you're capable yet.
    b. You want to go out with the gang for an evening on the town; your parents feel you should stay at home.

34. Use the following in a role-playing situation: Describe to a new friend what your eye problem is, when it started, how much you can see, and what is in store for the future (1, 3, 7).

35. From the biographical or autobiographical anecdotes quoted in this book, find an illustration of a problem situation or dilemma related to blindness. Read this to the group, stopping before the solution is given. Have the group provide possible solutions, then read the conclusion of the episode (1, 3, 7).

36. Identify the factors or events that help to produce

good or positive feelings and those that help to produce poor or negative feelings. What can be done to increase the likelihood of the former? to decrease the likelihood of the latter? (1, 3).

37. Discuss the problems involved in (a) overprotection (b) dependency, (c) self-acceptance, (d) fluctuating vision, and (e) ego-centrism (3, 7).

38. Role play the types of assistance offered and assistance received (discussed in Chapter 9), e.g. one plays the role of the Forceful Dominator, while the other plays the role of the Superindependent Refuser. Be sure to reverse roles (1, 6, 7).

39. Using a stop clock or cassette timed for two minutes, have the visually impaired person list as many "I can't" statements as he can in the two minute time period. At another time repeat the procedure for "I can" statements. Then compare the two lists (1, 4, 8).

40. Discuss the difference between praise and flattery. Identify a praise statement and a flattery statement regarding each member of the group. Have participants share their reactions to each statement (3).

41. Use Anagram™ tiles; words that describe or apply to self are "safe," cannot be stolen. Variation: Play Scrabble™; when a word applies or describes self, it is a "triple word" (4).

42. "How I feel about myself shows in how I behave." Have each group member give three illustrations of this principle (1, 3).

43. Have the participants list three joys experienced during each of the following age levels in their lives: preschool, primary, intermediate, junior high, senior high school. Variation: list three difficulties experienced during each age (2, 4).

44. Ask three members to participate in a discussion regarding a given topic, but secretly assign two of them to begin excluding the third. Afterward, have the third member share his feelings about being excluded. Discuss reactions of those who constantly feel rejected.

Speculate regarding some reasons for being excluded (5, 6).

45. What reactions do group members have to the idea discussed in Section II that lasting self-esteem emerges not so much from what a person has or does but rather from being part of God's creation (1, 8).

46. Ask members of the group to write the answers to these questions: What would you like to be doing five years from now? What will enable you to get there? Have them share their responses (4, 8).

47. For the next two days have each participant list his activities by 15 minute segments. After this is completed, have him decide which activities were characterized by others helping him, which by the participant helping himself, and which by the participant helping another (1, 2).

48. Assist group members to develop their self-esteem charts by having them pick a time period (10, 5, 1 year) and divide a piece of paper horizontally into distinct time periods. Number along the left margin from 10 to 1 (10 being high, 1 being low). Have each member plot his "self-esteem temperature" during each of the time periods and explain to a friend what contributed to each of the highs and each of the lows (2, 4).

49. Discuss the feelings a person has when he finds it necessary to ask for assistance from a family member? from a friend? from a stranger? Identify the factors that made one situation more difficult than another and discuss ways to make it easier (3, 7, 8).

50. Encourage participants to develop two lists: accomplishable goals and goals that are not accomplishable. See if other members of the group can suggest ways to reach goals thought to be unattainable (1, 8).

51. Ask each participant to make three lists: responsibilities that have been well-managed, responsibilities that have been poorly done, responsibilities that have been avoided. Discuss people's feelings about items on each list (2, 4).

52. Ask the participants to rank the following list of values in order of importance as guiding principles in their lives (1, 2): Inner harmony, Health, Self-respect, Beauty, Friendship, Social recognition, Self-sufficiency, Sense of accomplishment, Wisdom, Athletics or sports, Financial independence, Pleasure, Mature love, Status, Work, Body whole, Happiness, Food, Service to others, Humility, Personal rights, Moral conduct, Excitement, Normality.

53. Develop a file of newspaper clippings about blindness. From time to time read one to your group for their reactions. Can they determine whether the article emphasizes the succumbing or coping aspects of blindness, whether it tends to elicit pity or respect (3, 7).

54. Have the group discuss in what ways the adjusting process described in Chapter 8 applies to other types of trauma, such as divorce, death, loss of job (1).

55. As a group, read a biography of a visually impaired person (noted in the references with an asterisk) and provide time for the sharing of reactions. Identify some of the adjusting phases experienced by the visually impaired person and discuss the factors that enhanced or inhibited that adjusting process (1, 7).

BIBLIOGRAPHY

NOTE: Biography or autobiography of a visually impaired person indicated with asterisk.

Abel, G. L.: Adolescence: foothold on the future. *New Outlook, 55*: 103-106, 1961.

Acton, J.: Establishing and maintaining a therapeutic environment in a residential rehabilitation center for the blind. *New Outlook, 70*: 149-152, 1976.

Adler, A.: *Practice and Theory of Individual Psychology*, 2nd ed. London, Routledge, 1950.

Alley, S.: *100 Helps for Teachers*. Provo, Brigham Young University Press, 1978.

Allport, G.: *Personality: A Psychological Interpretation*. New York, Holt, Rinehart and Winston, 1937.

Argyris, C.: *Organization and Innovation*. Homewood, Il., Richard D. Irwin, 1965.

Arkoff, A.: *Adjustment and Mental Health*. New York, McGraw-Hill, 1968.

Asenjo, J., Project Director: *Rehabilitation Teaching for the Blind and Visually Disabled, the State of the Art*. New York, American Foundation for the Blind, 1975.

Baker, L.D.: Blindness and social behavior: a need for research. *New Outlook, 67*:315-318, 1973.

Barker, G., Wright, B.A., Meyerson, L., and Gonick, M.R.: *Adjustment to Physical Handicap and Illness: A Survey of the Social Psychology of Physique and Disability*. New York, Social Science Research Council, 1953.

*Barnes, E.W. *The Man Who Lived Twice: The Biography of Edward Sheldon*, N.Y., Scribner, 1956.

Barraga, N.: *Program to Develop Efficiency in Visual Functioning*. Louisville, Ky., Am. Printing House, 1980.

Barraga. N.: *Visual Handicaps and Learning: A Developmental Approach*. Belmont, Ca., Wadsworth, 1976.

297

Barron, S.: Cause of blindness and its impact on adjustment. Doctoral dissertation, City Univerity of N.Y., 1973.

*Barry, H.: *I'll Be Seeing you.* N.Y., Knopf, 1962.

Bateman, B.: Sighted children's perception of blind children's abilities. *Exceptional Children, 29*:42-46, 1962.

Bauman, M.K.: *Adjustment to Blindness.* Harrisburg, Pa. State Council for the Blind, 1954a.

Bauman, M.K.: Dimensions of blindness. In Goldberg, M. and Swinton, J. (Eds.): *Blindness Research: the Expanding Frontier.* University Park, Pa. State U. Press, 1969.

Bauman, M.K.: Group differences disclosed by inventory items. *International Journal for Ed. of the Blind, 13*:101-106, 1964.

Bauman, M.K.: The initial psychological reaction to blindness. *New Outlook, 53*:165-169, 1959.

Bauman, M.K.: A measure of personality change through adjustment training. *New Outlook, 48*:31-34, 1954b.

Bauman, M.K., and Yoder, N.: *Placing the Blind and Visually Handicapped in Professional Occupations.* Washington, D.C., U.S. Department of Health, Education and Welfare, 1962.

Benton, P.C.: The emotional aspects of visual handicaps. *Sight Saving Review, 21*:23-26, 1951.

*Bernstein, B.: *Thurber, A Biography.* N.Y., Dodd, Mead, 1975.

*Billington, M.L.: *Thomas P. Gore: The Blind Senator from Oklahoma.* Lawrence, University of Kansas Press, 1967.

*Blackhall, D.S.: *This House Had Windows.* N.Y., Obolensky, 1962.

*Blackhall, D.S.: *The Way I See it.* London, Baker, 1971.

Blank, H.R.: Psychoanalysis and blindness. *Psychoanalytic Quarterly, 26*:1-24, 1957.

Blank. H.R.: Reactions to loss of body parts—some research priorities in rehabilitation. *New Outlook, 62*:137-143, 1968.

Blechman, R.O.: *What Do You Do When You See a Blind Person?* N.Y., American Foundation for the Blind, 1970.

Block, J., and Thomas H.: Is satisfaction with self a measure of adjustment? *Journal of Abnormal Social Psychology, 51*(2):254-259, 1955.

*Boswell, C: *Now I See.* N.Y., Meredith Press, 1969.

*Bowen, B.: *Blind Man's Offering.* Boston, B. Bowen, 1947.

Bower, E.M.: The achievement of competency. In *Mental Health and Learning.* Washington, D.C., Association for Supervision and Curriculum Development, 1966.

Branden, N.: *The Psychology of Self-Esteem: A New Concept of Man's Psychological Nature.* Los Angeles, Nash, 1969.

*Bretz, A.: *I Begin Again.* N.Y., McGraw-Hill, 1940.

*Brown, E.G.: *Corridors of Light.* Yellow Springs, Oh, Antioch, 1958.

*Buckingham, T.H.: *Blind Educator: The Story of Newel Lewis Perry.* Berkeley, Ca., L. Buckingham, 1974.

Buell, C.E.: *Physical Education for Blind Children.* Springfield, Thomas, 1966.

Buell, C.E.: *Recreation for the Blind.* N.Y., American Foundation for the Blind, 1951.

Burlingham, D.: Some notes on the development of the blind. *Psychoanalytic Study of the Child, 16*:121-145, 1961.

Burlingham, D.: Some problems of ego development in blind children. *Psychoanalytic Study of the Child, 20*:194-208, 1965.

Burlingham, D.: To be blind in a sighted world. *Psychoanalytic Study of the Child, 34*:5-30, 1979.

*Campbell, M.: *No Compromise: The Story of Colonel Baker.* Toronto, McClelland and Steward, 1965.

Canfield, J., and Wells, H.: *100 Ways to Enhance Self-Concept in the Classroom.* Englewood Cliffs, Prentice-Hall, 1976.

Carroll, T.J.: *Blindness: What It Is, What It Does, and How To Live with It.* Boston, Little, Brown, 1961.

Carter, M.J., and Kelley, J.: Recreation programming for visually impaired children. In Kelley, J. (Ed.): *Recreation Programming for Visually Impaired Children and Youth.* N.Y., American Foundation for the Blind, 1981.

*Carver, S.: *A Girl and Five Brave Horses.* Garden City, N.Y., Doubleday, 1961.

*Caulfield, G.: *The Kingdom Within.* N.Y., Harper, 1960.

Chapman, E.K.: *Visually Handicapped Children and Young People.* London, Routledge, 1978.

*Charles, R., and Ritz, D.: *Brother Ray, Ray Charles' Own Story.* N.Y., Warner Books, 1978.

*Chevigny, H.: *My Eyes Have a Cold Nose.* New Haven, Yale University Press, 1946.

Chevigny, H., and Braverman, S.: *The Adjustment of the Blind.*New Haven, Yale University Press, 1950.

*Ching, L.: *One of the Lucky Ones.* Garden City, Doubleday, 1982.

Cholden, L.S.: *A Psychiatrist Works with Blindness.* New York, American Foundation for the Blind, 1958.

*Clark, E.: *Eyes, Etc.: A Memoir.* N.Y., Pantheon, 1977.

Clark. J.I.: *Self-Esteem, a Family Affair.* Minneapolis, Winston, 1978.

*Clifton, B.: *None So Blind.* Chicago, Rand McNally, 1963.

*Cline, H.: *William Hickling Prescott: A Memorial.* Durham, Duke University Press, 1959.

Coburn, H.H.: The psychological concept of dependency. *Rehabilitation Record, 5*:37-40, 1964.

Cohn, N.K.: Understanding the process of adjustment to disability. *Journal of Rehabilitation, 27*(6):16-18, 1961.

Coker, G.: A comparison of self-concepts and academic achievement of visually handicapped children enrolled in a regular school and in a residential school. *Education of the Visually Handicapped, 11*:67-76, 1979.

Combs, A.W., Soper, D.W., and Courson, C.C.: Measurement of self-concept and self report. *Educational and Psychological Measurement,* *23*:493-500, 1963.

Cook-Clampert, D.: The development of self-concept in blind children. *Visual Impairment and Blindness, 75*(6):237-238, 1981.

Cooley, C.H.: *Human Nature and the Social Order.* N.Y., Scribner, 1902.

Coopersmith, S. *The Antecedents of Self-esteem.* San Francisco, Freeman, 1967.

*Cordellos, H.: *Breaking Through.* Mountain View, Anderson, 1981.

Cowen, E.L., Underberg, R.P., Verrillo, R.T., and Benham, F.G.: *Adjustment of Visual Disability in Adolescence.* N.Y., American Foundation for the Blind, 1961.

Crandell, J.M., and Streeter, L.: The social adjustment of blind students in different educational settings. *Education of the Visually Handicapped 9*:1-7, 1977.

Cratty, B.J., and Sams, T.A.: *The Body Image of Blind Children.* N.Y., American Foundation for the Blind, 1968.

*Criddle, R.: *Love Is Not Blind.* N.Y., Norton, 1953.

Cull, J., and Hardy, E.: *Vocational Rehabilitation: Profession and Process.* Springfield, Thomas, 1972.

Cutsforth, T.D.: *The Blind in School and Society.* N.Y., American Foundation for the Blind, 1951, 1933.

Cutsforth, T.D.: Personality and social adjustment among the blind. In Zahl, P. (Ed.): *Blindness.* N.Y., Hafner, 1963, 1950.

*Dahl, B.: *Finding My Way.* N.Y., Dutton, 1962.

*Dahl, B.: *I Wanted to See.* N.Y., Macmillan, 1944.

Davies, C.: Three patterns of adjustment. *New Beacon, 51*(601):114-119, 1967.

Davis, C.J.: Development of the self-concept. *New Outlook, 58*:49-51, 1964.

*Degering, E. *Seeing Fingers. The Story of Louis Braille.* N.Y., McKay, 1962.

Delafield, G.L.: Adjustment to blindness. *Outlook for the Blind, 70*: 64-68, 1976.

De-Levie, A.: Attitudes of laymen and professions toward physical and social disability. Doctoral dissertation, Columbia University, 1966.

DeLoach, C., and Greer, B.: *Adjustment to Severe Disability: A Metamorphosis.* N.Y., McGraw-Hill, 1981.

Dinkmeyer, D.: *Developing Understanding of Self and Others (DUSO).* Circle Pines, Mn., American Guidance Service, 1970.

Dishart, M.: Family adjustment in the rehabilitation plan. *New Outlook, 58*:292-294, 1964.

Dobson, J.: *Hide or Seek.* Old Tappan, N.J., Revell, 1974.

Dobson, J.: *Preparing for Adolescence.* Santa Ana, Vision, 1978.

Dobson, J.: *Thirty Critical Problems Facing Today's Family.* Waco, Word, 1981.

Dobson, J.: *What Wives Wish Their Husbands Knew About Women.*

Wheaton, Tyndale, 1975.

Dover, F.: Readjusting to the onset of blindness. *Social Casework, 40*: 334-338, 1959.

Dupont, H., Gardner, O.S., and Brody, D.: *Toward Affective Development.* Circle Pines, Mn., American Guidance Association, 1974.

Duval, S., and Wicklund, R.A.: *A Theory of Objective Self-Awareness.* New York, Academic Press, 1972.

*Edwards, G.: *Keep in Touch.* London, MacGibbon & Kee, 1962.

Eisenstadt, A.A.: Psychological problems of the parents of a blind child. *Int J Educ Blind, 5*(1):20-24, 1955.

Emerson, D.: Facing loss of vision: the response of adults to visual impairment and blindness. *Journal of Visual Impairment and Blindness, 75*(2):41-45, 1981.

Erikson, E.H.: *Childhood and Society.* N.Y., Norton, 1950.

Everhart, G.: Assertive skills training for the blind. *Journal of Visual Impairment and Blindness, 74*:62-65, 1980.

*Fawcett, M.G.: *What I Remember.* T.F., Unwin, 1925.

Festinger, L.: *A Theory of Cognitive Dissonance.* Stanford, Stanford University Press, 1962.

Fitting, E.A.: Analysis of factors relating to adjustment to blindness. Doctoral dissertation, Michigan State U., 1957.

Fitting, E.A.: *An Evaluation of Adjustment to Blindness.* N.Y., American Foundation for the Blind, 1954.

Fitts, W.H.: *Interpersonal Competence: The Wheel Model.* Nashville, Counselor Recordings and Tests, 1970.

Fitts, W.H.: *The Self Concept and Behavior, Overview and Supplement.* Nashville, Dede Wallace Center, 1972.

Fitts, W.H.: *The Self Concept as a Variable in Vocational Rehabilitation.* Nashville, Mental Health Center, 1967.

Fitzgerald, R.G.: Reactions to blindness: an exploratory study of adults with recent loss of sight. *Archives of General Psychiatry, 22*:370-379, 1970.

Fitzgerald, R.G.: Visual phenomenology in recently blind adults. *American Journal of Psychiatry, 127*(11):109-115, 1971.

Foulke, E.: The personality of the blind: a non-valid concept. *New Outlook,66*(2):33-37, 42, 1972.

*Fox, M.L.: *Blind Adventure.* N.Y., Lippincott, 1946.

Fraiberg, S.: *Insights from the Blind.*Ann Arbor, University of Michigan Press, 1977.

Fraiberg, S., and Adelson, E.: Self representation in young blind children. In Zofjas, J. (Ed.): *On the Effects of Blindness and Other Impairments on Early Development.* N.Y., American Foundation for the Blind, 1976.

*Frank, M.: *First Lady of the Seeing Eye.* N.Y., Holt, Rinehart and Winston, 1957.

302   *Self-Esteem and Adjusting with Blindness*

*Fraser, I.: *Whereas I Was Blind.* London, Hodder & Stoughton, 1946.
Freed, A.: *TA for Teens and Other Important People.* Sacramento, Jalmar, 1976.
*Fries, E.B.: *But You Can Feel It.* Portland, Binford & Mort, 1980.
Fromm, E.: *Man for Himself, An Inquiry into the Psychology of Ethics.* N.Y., Holt, Rinehart and Winston, 1947.
Fromm, E.: Selfishness and self-love. *Psychiatry: Journal for the Study of Interpersonal Processes,* 2:507-523, 1939.
Galler, E.H.: A long-term support group for elderly people with low vision. *Journal of Visual Impairment and Blindness,* 75:173-176, 1981.
Gardner, L.: Understanding and helping parents of blind children. *Journal of Visual Impairment and Blindness,* 76(3):81-85, 1982.
Gearheart, B.R.: *Special Education for the '80's.* St. Louis, Mosby, 1980.
Gergan, K.J.: *The Concept of Self.* N.Y., Holt, Rinehart and Winston, 1971.
Giarratana-Oehler, J.: Personal and professional reactions to blindness from diabetic retinopathy. *New Outlook,* 70:237-239, 1976.
Goffman, E.: *Stigma.* Englewood Cliffs, Prentice Hall, 1963.
Gomulicki, B.R.: *The Development of Perception and Learning in Blind Children.* University of Cambridge Psychological Laboratory, 1961.
Greenberg, H.M.: *Teaching with Feeling: Compassion and Self-Awareness in the Classroom Today.* N.Y., Macmillan, 1969.
Greenough, T.J., Keegan, D.L, and Ash, D.G.: Psychological and social adjustment of blind subjects on the 16 PF. *Journal of Clinical Psychology,* 34(1):84-87, 1978.
Halliday, C.: *The Visually Inpaired Child: Growth, Learning, Development, Infancy to School Age.* Louisville, American Printing House for the Blind, 1970.
Hamachek, D.E.: *Encounters with the Self.* N.Y., Holt, Rinehart and Winston, 1971.
Hardy, R.E., and Cull, J.G.: *Social and Rehabilitation Services for the Blind.* Springfield, Thomas, 1972.
Harley, R.K.: Children with visual disabilities. In Dunn, L. (Ed.): *Exceptional Children in the Schools.* N.Y., Holt, Rinehart and Winston, 1973.
Harshberger, C.: Group work with elderly visually impaired persons. *Journal of Visual Impairment and Blindness,* 74(6):221-224, 1980.
*Hartman, D. & Asbell, B.: *White Coat, White Cane,* Chicago, Playboy, 1978.
*Haskins, J.: *The Story of Stevie Wonder.* N.Y., Lothrop Lee and Shepard, 1976.
Hatfield, E.M.: Why are they blind? *Sight Saving Review.* 45:3-22, 1975.
Head, D.: A comparison of self-concept scores for visually impaired adolescents in several class settings. *Education of the Visually Handicapped,* 10:51-55, 1979.

*Henderson, L.T.: *The Opening Doors: My Child's First Eight Years without Sight.* N.Y., John Day, 1954.

Hey, C.: Social aspects of becoming visually impaired in later life: a study in the socialization with visual impairment. Doctoral dissertation, Boulder, U. of Colorado, 1981.

*Hickford, J.: *Eyes at my Feet.* N.Y., St. Martin's, 1973.

*Hickford, J.: *I Never Walked Alone.* N.Y., St. Martin's, 1977.

Hicks, S.: Psycho-social and rehabilitation aspects of acquired visual handicap. *New Beacon, 63*(747):169-174, 1979.

*Hocken, S.: *Emma and I.* N.Y., Dutton, 1978.

*Hogg, G.: *Blind Jack of Knaresborough: Road Builder Extraordinary.* London: Phoenix House, 1967.

*Holmes, C.S.: *The Clocks of Columbus: The Literary Career of James Thurber,* N.Y., Atheneum, 1972.

Horney, K.: *Our Inner Conflicts.* N.Y., Norton, 1945.

*Husing, E. and Lewis, J.: *My Eyes Are My Heart.* N.Y., B. Geis, 1959.

*Irwin, R.B.: *As I Saw It.* N.Y., American Foundation for the Blind, 1955.

James. W.: *Principles of Psychology.* N.Y., Holt, 1890.

Jan, J., Scott, E.P., and Freeman, R.: *Visual Impairment in Children and Adolescents.* N.Y., Grune and Stratton, 1977.

Jervis, F.M.: A comparison of self concepts of blind and sighted children. In Davis, C.J. (Ed.): *Guidance Programs for Blind Children.* Watertown, Ma., Perkins, 1959.

Jervis, F.M.: The self in process of obtaining and maintaining self-esteem. *New Outlook, 58*:51-54, 1964.

Jervis, F.M., and Haslerud, G.M.: Qualitative and quantitative differences in frustration between blind and sighted adolescents. *Readings on the Exceptional Child.* N.Y., Appleton Century-Crofts, 1962.

Jones, R.L., Gottfried, N.W., and Owens, A.: The social distance of the exceptional: a study at the high school level. *Exceptional Children, 32*:551-557, 1966.

Jones, W.P.: Identifying minimum coping competencies for visually impaired. *Education of the Visually Handicapped, 12*:4-10, 1980.

Jourard, S.M.: Healthy personality and self-disclosure. *Mental Hygiene, 43*:499-506, 1959.

Jourard, S.M.: *Personal Adjustment: An Approach Through the Study of Healthy Personality.* N.Y., Macmillan, 1963.

Kappan, D.: Orientation and mobility. In *Handbook for Teachers of the Visually Impaired.* Louisville, American Printing House for the Blind, 1981.

*Keitlen, T.: *Farewell to Fear.* N.Y., B. Geis, 1960.

Kelley, J. (Ed.): *Recreation Programming for the Visually Impaired Children and Youth.* N.Y., American Foundation for the Blind, 1981.

*Kemper, R.G.: *An Elephant's Ballet: One Man's Successful Struggle with*

Sudden Blindness. N.Y., Seabury, 1977.

Kirchner, C., and Peterson, R.: Statistical brief # 9. *Journal of Visual Impairment and Blindness, 74*(5):203-205, 1980.

Kirchner, C., and Peterson, R.: Statistical brief #15. *Journal of Visual Impairment and Blindness, 74*(5):267-270, 1981.

Kirtley, D.D.: *The Psychology of Blindness.* Chicago, Nelson-Hall, 1975.

Kizziar, J.: *Search for Acceptance: The Adolescent and Self-esteem.* Chicago, Nelson-Hall, 1979.

Klein, G.S.: Blindness and isolation. *Psychoanalytic Study of the Child. 17:*82-93, 1962.

Klich, B., and Wierig, G.J.: Social interaction and emotional adjustment among the blind. *Percept Motor Skills, 32:*516-518, 1971.

*Krents, H.: *To Race the Wind.* N.Y., Putnam, 1972.

Kübler-Ross, E.: *On Death and Dying.* N.Y., Macmillan, 1969.

Kurzhals, I.W.: Personality adjustment for the blind child in the classroom. *New Outlook, 64*(5):129-134, 1970.

LaBenne, W., and Greene, B.I.: *Educational Implications of Self-concept Theory.* Pacific Palisades, Goodyear, 1969.

Lambert, R.M., West, M., and Carlin, K.: Psychology of adjustment to visual deficiency: a conceptual model. *Journal of Visual Impairment and Blindness, 75:*193-196, 1981.

Land, S.L, and Vineberg, S.E.: Locus of control in blind children. *Exceptional Children, 31:*257-260, 1965.

Lazarus, R.S.: *Patterns of Adjustment.* N.Y., McGraw-Hill, 1969.

Locke, D., and Gerler, E. Psychological education for visually impaired children. *Education fo the Visually Handicapped, 11:*118-120, 1979.

Locke, D., and Gerler, E.: Affective education for visually impaired children. *Humanist Educator,* 20:11-20, 1981.

Lowenfeld, B.: *Berthold Lowenfeld on Blindness and Blind People. Selected Papers.* N.Y., American Foundation for the Blind, 1981.

Lowenfeld, B.: *The Changing Status of the Blind from Separation to Integration.* Springfield, Thomas, 1975.

Lowenfeld, B.: *Our Blind Children, Growing and Learning with Them.* Springfield, Thomas, 1971a.

Lowenfeld, B.: Psychological foundations of special methods in teaching blind children. In Zahl, P.A. (Ed.):*Blindness.* N.Y., Hafner, 1963, 1950.

Lowenfeld, B.: Psychological problems of children with impaired vision. In Cruickshank, W. (Ed.): *Psychology of Exceptional Children.* Englewood Cliffs, Prentice Hall, 1971b, 1980.

Lowenfeld, B.: *The Visually Handicapped Child in School.* N.Y., John Day, 1973.

Lowenfeld, B., Abel, G.L., and Hatlen, P.: *Blind Children Learn to Read.* Springfield, Thomas, 1969.

Lukoff, I., and Cohen, O. (Eds.): *Attitudes Toward Blind Persons.* N.Y., American Foundation for the Blind, 1972.

Lukoff, I., and Whiteman, M.: *The Social Sources of Adjustment to Blindness.* N.Y., American Foundation for the Blind, 1970.

*Lunt, L: *If You Make a Noise I Can't See.* London, Gollancz, 1965.

*Lusseyran, J.: *And There Was Light.* Boston, Little, Brown, 1963.

Lyndon, W.T., and McGraw, M.L.: *Concept Development for Visually Handicapped Children.* N.Y., American Foundation for the Blind, 1973.

Mangold, S.S.: Nurturing high self-esteem in visually handicapped children. In Mangold, S.S. (Ed.): *A Teacher's Guide to the Special Educational Needs of Blind and Visually Handicapped Children.* N.Y., American Foundation for the Blind, 1982.

Maslow, A.H.: *Motivation and Personality.* New York, Harper and Row, 1954, 1970.

Mayadas, N.S.: Role expectations and performance of blind children: practice and implications. *Education of the Visually Handicapped, 4:* 45-52, 1972.

Mayadas, N.S., and Duehn, W.D.: The impact of significant adult's expectations on the life style of visually impaired children. *New Outlook, 70:*286-290, 1976.

McAndrew, H.: Rigidity and isolation: a study of the deaf and the blind. *Journal of Abnormal Social Psychology, 43:*476-494, 1948.

McCandless, B.R.: *Children: Behavior and Development.* New York, Holt, Rinehart and Winston, 1967, 1977.

*McCoy, M.B.: *Journey Out of Darkness.* N.Y., McKay, 1963.

Mead, G.H.: *Mind, Self and Society.* Chicago, University of Chicago, 1934.

*Mehta, V.: *Daddyji.* N.Y., Farrar, Straus, Giroux, 1972.

*Mehta, V.: *Face to Face.* Boston, Little, Brown, 1957.

Meighan, T. *An Investigation of the Self Concept of Blind and Visually Handicapped Adolescents.* N.Y., American Foundation for the Blind, 1971.

Meyerson, L.: Somatopsychology of physical disability. In Cruickshank, W. (Ed.): *Psychology of Exceptional Children and Youth.* Englewood Cliffs, Prentice-Hall, 1971.

Miller, W.H.: Group counseling with the blind. *Education of the Visually Handicapped, 3:*46-51, 1971.

Miller, W.H.: Manifest anxiety in visually impaired adolescents. *Education of the Visually Handicapped, 2:*91-95, 1970.

*Minton, H.G.: *Blind Man's Buff.* London, England, Elek, 1974.

*Mitchell, M.: *Uncharted Country, Aspects of Life in Blindness.* Melbourne, Longman Cheshire, 1964.

Monbeck, M.E.: *The Meaning of Blindness.* Bloomington, Indiana University Press, 1973.

*Moore, V.B.: *Seeing Eye Wife.* Philadelphia, Chilton, 1960.

Moos, R.H., and Tsu, V.D.: The crisis of physical illness. In Moos, R.H.

(Ed.): *Coping with Physical Illness*. N.Y., Plenum, 1977.

*Morgan, B.K.: *Obstacle Course*. San Francisco, Chronicle, 1979.

Morse, W.C., Ardizzonne, J., MacDonald, C., and Pasick, P. *Affective Education for Special Children and Youth*. Reston, Council for Exceptional Children, 1980.

Mussen, P.H., and Newman, D.K.: Acceptance of handicap, motivation and adjustment in physically disabled children. *Exceptional Children*, 24:255-260, 277-279, 1959.

Napier, G.: Special subject adjustments and skills. In Lowenfeld, B. (Ed.): *The Visually Handicapped Child in School*. N.Y., John Day, 1973.

National Society to Prevent Blindness: *Vision Problems in the U.S.* New York, National Society to Prevent of Blindness, 1980.

*Nauman, A.: *Flame in the Dark*. London, Collins, 1962.

Needham, W.E., and Ehmer, M.H.: Irrational thinking and adjustment to loss of vision. *Journal of Visual Impairment and Blindness*, 74 (2):57-61, 1980.

Neu, C.: Coping with newly diagnosed blindness. *American Journal of Nursing*, 75(12):2161-2163, 1975.

Norris, M., Spaulding, P.J., and Brodie, F.H.: *Blindness in Children*. Chicago, University of Chicago Press, 1957.

Oehler-Giarratana, J., and Fitzgerald, R.: Group therapy with blind diabetics. *Archives of General Psychiatry*, 37 (4):463-467, 1980.

*Ohnstad, K.: *The World at My Finger Tips*. N.Y., Bobbs-Merrill, 1942.

Palomares, U., and Ball, G.: *Human Development Program*. "The Magic Circle." LaMesa, Human Development Training Institute, 1972.

Parad, H.J., and Caplan, G.: A framework for studying families in crisis. In Parad, H. (Ed.): *Crisis Intervention*. N.Y., Family Service Association, 1965.

Parkes, C.M.: *Bereavement: Studies of Grief in Adult Life*. New York, International Universities Press, 1972.

*Patterson, G.D.: *The Strawberry Apple Tree*. San Antonio, Naylor, 1971.

Pearlman, J.T., Adams, G.L., and Sloan, S.H.: *Psychiatric Problems in Ophthalmology*. Springfield, Thomas, 1977.

*Perry, E., and Roy, F.H.: *Light in the Shadows: Feelings about Blindness*. Little Rock, World Eye Foundation, 1982.

*Pierce, R.: *It Was Not My Own Idea*. N.Y., American Foundation for the Blind, 1944.

*Potok, A.: *Ordinary Daylight: Portrait of an Artist Going Blind*. N.Y., Holt, Rinehart and Winston, 1980.

*Putnam, P.: *Cast off the Darkness*. N.Y., Harcourt, Brace, 1957.

*Putnam, P.: *"Keep Your Head Up, Mr. Putnam!"* N.Y., Harper, 1952.

Rapp, D.W.: *The Developmental Nature of Self-Concept*. Hattiesburgh, Miss., Bureau of Educational Research, University of Southern Miss., 1974.

Resnick, R.: The relationship between self-concept, independence and the life styles of congenitally blind persons in terms of integration. Doctoral dissertation. University of San Francisco, 1981.

*Resnick, R.: *Sun and Shadow.* N.Y., Atheneum, 1975.

*Richard, C.: *Climbing Blind.* N.Y., Dutton, 1967.

Riffenburgh, R.: The psychology of blindness. *Geriatrics, 22*:127-133, 1967.

Roberts, A.: *Psychosocial Rehabilitation of the Blind.* Springfield, Thomas, 1973.

*Robinson, L.A.: *Light at the Tunnel End.* Silver Springs, Md., Foundation for Handicapped and Elderly, 1975.

*Roblin, J.: *The Reading Fingers: Life of Louis Braille.* New York, American Foundation for the Blind, 1955.

Roessler, R., and Boone, S.E.: Locus of control, self-esteem, and hope for individuals with visual impairments. *Rehabilitation Counseling Bulletin, 22*:448-450, 1979.

Rogers, C.: *Client Centered Therapy: Its Current Practice, Implications and Theory.* Boston, Houghton Mifflin, 1951.

Rogers, C.: *On Becoming a Person.* Boston, Houghton Mifflin, 1961.

Rogers, C.: Personality and interpersonal relationships. In Koch, S. (Ed.): *Psychology: A Study of a Science,* Vol III. New York, McGraw-Hill, 1959.

Rosenberg, M.: *Society and the Adolescent Self-image.* Princeton, Princeton University Press, 1965.

Routh, T.: *Rehabilitation Counseling of the Blind.* Springfield, Thomas, 1970.

*Ruffin, B.: *Fanny Crosby.* Philadelphia, United Church Press, 1976.

Rusalem, H.: *Coping with the Unseen Environment.* N.Y., Teachers College Press, Columbia University, 1972.

*Russell, R.: *The Island.* N.Y., Vangaurd, 1973.

*Russell, R.: *To Catch an Angel.* N.Y., Vanguard, 1962.

*Ruuth, M.: *Stevie Wonder.* Los Angeles, Holloway House, 1980.

Safilios-Rothschild, C.: *The Sociology and Social Psychology of Disability and Rehabilitation.* N.Y., Random, 1970.

Samuels, S.: *Enhancing Self-concept in Early Childhood: Theory and Practice.* N.Y., Human Sciences Press, 1977.

*Sanford, C.: *Second Sight.* N.Y., Evans, 1979.

Schindele, R.: Social adjustment of visually handicapped in different educational settings. *Research Bulletin #28,* N.Y., American Foundation for the Blind, 1974.

Scholl, G.T.: Affective Competencies of Teachers of Visually Handicapped Students: Identification and Development. Reston, Va., Council for Exceptional Children, 1982.

Scholl, G.T.: Understanding and meeting developmental needs. In Lowenfeld, B. (Ed.): *The Visually Handicapped Child in School.*

N.Y., John Day, 1973.

Scholl, G.T., Bauman, M.K., and Crissey, M.S.: *A Study of the Vocational Success of Groups of the Visually Handicapped.* Ann Arbor, University of Michigan, 1969.

Schulz, P.: *How Does It Feel to be Blind?* Van Nuys, Ca., Muse-Ed, 1980.

Scott, E.P., Jan, J., and Freeman, R.: *Can't Your Child See?* Baltimore, University Park Press, 1977.

Scott, R.A.: *The Making of Blind Men: A Study of Adult Socialization.* N.Y., Russell Sage Foundation, 1969a.

Scott, R.A.: Socialization of blind children. In Goslin, D. (Ed.): *Handbook of Socialization Theory and Research.* N.Y., Rand McNally, 1969b.

Secord, P.F., and Jourard, S.M.: The appraisal of body cathexis: body cathexis and the self. *Journal of Consulting Psychology, 17*:343-347, 1953.

Severson, A.L.: Adjustment to blindness. *New Outlook, 47*(3):81-82, 1953.

*Sewell, R., and G.: *House Without Windows.* Toronto, Martin, 1974.

Shaffer, L.F., and Shoben, E.J.: *The Psychology of Adjustment.* Boston, Houghton Mifflin, 1956.

*Sheppard, W.: *Out of My Darkness.* N.Y., Frederick Fell, 1956.

Siller, J, Ferguson, L., Vann, D., and Holland, B.: Structure of attitudes toward the physically disabled. In *Studies in Reactions to Disability XII.* N.Y., New York University, 1967.

Smith, C.: The relationship between self-concept and success in the freshman year of college. *New Outlook, 66*:84-89, 1972.

Smithdas, R.J.: *Psychological aspects of deaf-blindness.* Sands Point, N.Y., Helen Keller National Center for Deaf-Blind Youth and Adults. Reprinted from presentation at 1975 Convention of the World Federation of the Deaf.

Sommers, V.: *The Influence of Parental Attitudes and Social Environment on the Personality Development of Adolescent Blind.* N.Y., American Foundation for the Blind, 1944.

*Sperber, A.: *Out of Sight: Ten Stories of Victory over Blindness.* Boston, Little, Brown, 1976.

*Stainback, B.: *A Very Different Love Story.* N.Y., Morrow, 1977.

Steinzor, L.V.: Visually handicapped children: their attitudes toward blindness. *Outlook, 60*:307-311, 1966.

Stephens, W.B., and Grube, C.: Development of Piagetian reasoning in congenitally blind children. *Journal of Visual Impairment and Blindness, 76*(4):133-143, 1982.

Stephens, W.B., and Simpkins, K.: *The Reasoning, Moral Judgment and Moral Conduct of the Congenitally Blind.* Washington, D.C., U.S. Department of Health, Education and Welfare, 1974.

Stevens, J.O.: *Awareness: Exploring, Experimenting and Experiencing.* Des Plaines, Bantam, 1973.

Stogner, P.C.: The effects of typical retinitis pigmentosa, Leber's congenital amaurosis, centroperipheral dystrophy, and Usher's syndrome on
educational and vocational success and personality development.
International Journal of Rehabilitation Research, 3(3):357-366, 1980.

Stotland, E., and Canon, L.K.: *Social Psychology: A Cognitive Approach.*
Philadelphia, Saunders, 1972.

Stringer, L.A.: *A Sense of Self, A Guide to How We Mature.* Philadelphia,
Temple University Press, 1971.

Sullivan, H.S.: *The Interpersonal Theory of Psychiatry.* N.Y., Norton,
1953.

*Sullivan, T., and Gill, D.: *If You Could See What I Hear.* N.Y., Harper and
Row, 1975.

Suterko, S.: Life adjustment. In Lowenfeld, B. (Ed.): *The Visually Handicapped Child in School.* N.Y., John Day, 1973.

Swallow, R.: Piaget's theory and the visually handicapped child. *New
Outlook, 70*:273-281, 1976.

Symonds, P.M.: *The Ego and the Self.* N.Y., Appleton-Century-Crofts,
1951.

Thume, L., and Murphree, O.D.: Acceptance of the white cane and hope
for the restoration of sight in blind persons as an indicator of
adjustment. *Journal of Clinical Psychology, 17*(2):208-209, 1961.

*Thurber, J.: *My Life and Hard Times.* N.Y., Harper, 1933.

Trismen, D.A.: Equating braille forms of the sequential tests of educational progress. *Exceptional Children, 33*:419-424, 1967.

Tuttle, D.W.: Academics are not enough. In *Handbook for Teachers of the
Visually Impaired.* Louisville, American Printing House, 1981a, pp.
38-44.

Tuttle, D.W.: Audio reading: an effective alternative. In *Handbook for
Teachers of the Visually Impaired.* Louisville, American Printing
House, 1981b, pp. 26-37.

Tuttle, D.W.: A comparison of three reading media for the blind.
Education of Visually Handicapped, 4:40-44, 1972.

*Twersky, J.: *The Sound of the Walls.* Garden City, Doubleday, 1959.

*Ulrich, S.: *Elizabeth.* Ann Arbor, University of Michigan Press, 1972.

*Vajda, A.: *Journey Round My Eye.* England, Hutchinson, 1962.

*Vajda, A.: *Lend Me an Eye.* N.Y., St. Martin's, 1974.

VanderKolk, D.J.: *Assessment and Planning with the Visually Handicapped.* Baltimore, University Park Press, 1981.

Weinberg, J.R.: A further investigation of the body cathexis and the
self. *Journal of Consulting Psychology, 24*:277-281, 1960.

*Weller, R.: *Blind and I See!* St. Louis, Concordia, 1978.

Wells, L.E., and Marwell, G.: *Self-esteem, Its Conceptualization and
Measurement.* Beverly Hills, Sage, 1976.

Welsh, R.L.: Psychosocial dimensions. In Welsh, R.L., and Blasch, B.:
Foundations of Orientation and Mobility. N.Y., American Founda-

tion for the Blind, 1980.

Welsh, R.L.: The use of group strategies with the visually impaired. In Seligman, M. (Ed.): *Group Psychotherapy and Counseling with Special Populations.* Baltimore, University Park Press, 1982.

Wenkart, A.: The self and the process of integration. *American Journal of Psychoanalysis, 10*:91-92, 1950.

West, E.: My child is blind, thoughts on family life. *Exceptional Parent, 11*:9-12, 1981.

*Westrate, E.: *Beacon in the Night.* N.Y., Vantage, 1964.

Winton, C.A.: On the realization of blindness. *New Outlook, 64*:16-24, 1970.

Wright, B.A.: An analysis of attitudes—dynamics and effects. *New Outlook, 68*, 108-118, 1974.

Wright, B.A.: *Physical Disability-A Psychological Approach.* N.Y., Harper, 1960.

Wyder, F.T., Wilson, M.E., and Frumkin, R.M.: Information as a factor in perception of the blind by teachers. *Perceptual and Motor Skills, 25*:188, 1967.

Wylie, R.: *The Self Concept, A Critical Survey of Pertinent Research.* Lincoln, University of Nebraska Press, 1961.

Yank, B.: A new approach to adjustment training for blinded individuals. *New Outlook, 62*(10):313-318, 1968.

*Yates, E.: *The Lighted Heart.* N.Y., Dutton, 1960.

Younie, W., and Rusalem, H.: *The World of Rehabilitation: An Atlas for Special Educators.* N.Y., Day, 1971.

Zunich, M., and Ledwith, B.E.: Self-concepts of visually handicapped and sighted children. *Perceptual and Motor Skills, 21*:771-774, 1965.

*Zook, D.: *Debby.* Scottdale, Pa., Herald Press, 1974.

INDEX

A

Abel, G.L., xv, 52, 245
Acceptance, 155, 196, 202, 223-224
Acton, J., 147, 220
Adaptive behaviors, 203, 206-209, 209-213
Adjusting process, 54-56, 145-158, 283
    diagram, summary, 238
    factors influencing, 239-276
    models, 151-156, 159-238
Adjusting with blindness, xiv, 146, 156, 159-238, 288
    definition, 8, 231-238
Adjustment, 149-151, 154, 155, 197, 206, 228
    definition, 146-149
Adler, A., 67, 115, 137
Age at time of trauma, 161-162, 166, 244-247
Alley, S., 289
Allport, G., 62
Anger, 154, 155, 177, 182, 194, 220
Anxiety, 123
Argyris, C., 99
Arkoff, A., 128, 146
Asbell, B., 41, 42, 68, 69, 81, 89, 133, 134, 162, 172, 209, 245
Ash, D.G., 240
"As if" behavior, 131, 197, 248
Aspirations and goals, 73, 94-96, 107, 154, 190, 197-199, 282
Assets and strengths, 197-199, 203
Assimilation, 10, 12, 48, 81
Assistance, offered, 234, 267, 268-271
Assistance, received, 267, 271-275
Attitudes, of the blind, 160, 242, 288
Attitudes, social, 8-12, 45-49, 71, 72, 83-88, 208, 225, 243, 269
Attributes, defining (DA), 68-70, 79, 92, 118, 122, 125-126, 129-130
    discordant or harmonious, 73-76

Attributes, personal (PA), 68-70, 88, 92, 118, 122, 125, 126, 129, 130, 194, 197, 226, 288

B

Baker, L.D., 47
Ball, G., 289
Barker, G., 45
Barraga, N., 13, 16, 23
Barron, S., 251
Bateman, B., 48, 70
Bauman, M.K., 33, 56, 82, 146, 149, 151, 217, 244, 247
Benham, F.G., 56, 149, 151, 247, 257
Bernstein, B., 124, 132, 173
Bibliotherapy, 201, 219, 260, 293
Blackhall, D.S., 29, 32, 103, 161, 179, 181, 200, 202, 233, 275
Blank, H.R., 53, 147, 157, 162, 171, 187, 188, 206, 239, 240, 252, 263
Blasch, B., 25
Blechman, R.O., 280
Blindness
    acceptance of, 223-226, 288
    adventitious, 15, 21-22, 34, 36, 51, 157, 160-162, 167-169, 170, 196, 212, 259, 262
    assimilating implications of, 223-226
    congenital, 14, 21-22, 157, 160, 162-165, 168-169, 170, 195, 196, 242
    consequences of, 6, 18, 38-49
    definition, 12, 14-15
    incidence, 16-17
    prevalence, 16-17
    psychology of, 38, 147, 284
    (*see also* Visual loss; Low vision)
Boswell, C.A., 207, 213, 253, 281
Bower, E.M., 98
Braverman, S., 269
Bretz, A., 45, 105, 186, 200, 201, 207,

216, 220, 225, 227, 229, 240, 247, 253, 264
Brodie, F.H., 19
Brody, D., 289
Brown, E., 50, 135, 164, 170, 196
Buell, C.E., 37
Burlingham, D., 162

C

Canfield, J., 280, 284, 289
Canon, L.K., 99
Caplan, G., 210
Carlin, K., 149, 188, 207, 214
Carroll, T.J., 147, 184
Carter, M.J., 37
Carver, S., 12, 106, 172, 198, 230
Caulfield, G., 71, 87, 222
Chapman, E.K., 50, 111, 265
Charles, R., 96, 265
Chevigny, H., 45, 71, 72, 88, 174, 176, 197, 262, 263, 268, 269
Cholden, L.S., 48, 147, 148, 149, 153, 154, 171, 172, 173, 179, 187, 190, 196, 210, 226, 240, 242, 254
Clark, E., 168, 182, 195, 248, 250
Clifton, B., 22, 48, 77, 84, 171, 198
Coburn, H.H., 266
Cohen, O., 45
Cohn, N.K., 153, 157, 175, 182, 198, 214, 234
Coker, G., 57, 151
Combs, A.W., 65
Communication skills, 29-32
Competence, 99-100, 261
   model, 91-120
   model, diagram, 93, 119
Conceptualization, 49-52
Conflicts, 98, 106, 110, 114, 121-142
Confrontation, 174, 231, 232
Cook-Clampert, D., 66, 97, 256, 264
Cooley, C.H., 68, 115
Coopersmith, S., 63, 64, 82, 88, 92, 95, 96, 104, 105, 107, 111, 112, 127, 136, 137, 257, 264, 265
Coping, 85, 155, 205-223, 225, 234, 242, 263
Cordellos, H., 132, 208
Cowen, E.L., 56, 149, 151, 247, 256
Cratty, B.J., 67
Crissey, M.S., 33

Cutsforth, T.D., 41, 51, 152

D

Dahl, B., 21, 40, 46, 97, 108, 191, 203, 220, 242, 249, 257, 273
Daily living skills, 21-22
Davies, C., 232
Davis, C.J., 67, 247
Defense mechanisms, 136-137, 153, 154, 155, 170, 172-173, 175, 233
Defining attributes (DA) (*see* Attributes, defining)
Delafield, G.L., 61, 147, 149, 157, 279
DeLevie, A., 48
Deloach, C., 283
Denial (*see* Defense mechanisms)
Dependence, 19, 29, 41-43, 185, 240-241, 262-275
Depression, 153, 154, 155, 181, 186-189, 194, 240, 250
Developmental stages, 116-118
Dinkmeyer, D., 289
Disability, 13-14
Discrepancies, 98, 106, 110, 114
   resolution of, 121-142, 128-136, 163
Dishart, M., 255
Dissonance reduction, 75-76
   (*see also* Discrepancies, resolution of)
Dobson, J., 64, 120, 137, 186, 190, 284
Dog guide (*see* Orientation and mobility)
Dover, F., 153, 157, 188, 197, 206, 209, 240
Dupont, H., 289

E

Education, 10, 11, 280
   career, 34
Edwards, G., 24, 31, 32, 35, 36, 46, 84, 85, 100, 166, 202, 230, 262, 270, 274
Ehmer, M.H., 252
Egocentrism, 39-40, 176-177, 192
Eisenstadt, A.A., 256
Emerson, D., 149, 180, 184, 188, 192, 204, 240, 242
Employment, 32-35, 246, 259, 261-262, 279
Environment, physical and social, 76-78, 232, 242

Erikson, E.H., 115
Expectations, 94-95, 96-98, 107, 109, 211, 282

F

Failure, 107-111, 127, 220
Faith, 199-201, 252-253
Fear, 155, 176, 180, 246
Festinger, L., 122
Fitting, E.A., 149, 221
Fitts, W.H., 56, 63, 65, 82, 267, 275, 279, 284
Fitzgerald, R.G., 155, 157, 189, 199, 214, 249
Foulke, E., 38
Fox, M.L., 22, 44, 46, 167, 185, 192, 199, 200, 201, 219
Fraiberg, S., 66, 67
Freeman, R., 245, 255
Fries, E.B., 10, 21, 44, 46, 69, 95, 135, 235, 243, 247, 259
Fromm, E., 64, 65, 115, 229
Frumkin, R.M., 48

G

Galler, E.H., 204
Gardner, L., 255
Gardner, O.S., 289
Gearheart, B.R., 16
Gergan, K.J., 45, 62, 64, 73, 76, 80, 89, 95, 104, 109, 127, 128, 211
Gerler, E., 289
Giarratana-Oehler, J., 146, 156, 157, 193, 228, 250, 263
Gill, D., 41, 68, 85, 178, 183, 228, 273
Goals (*see* Aspirations and goals)
Goffman, E., 61, 132
Gomulicki, B.R., 265
Gonick, M.R., 45
Greene, B., 64, 68, 96, 104, 108, 111, 127, 145, 211, 280, 284
Greenough, T.J., 240
Group, support, 192, 204, 217-218, 287
Grube, C., 52

H

Halliday, C., 66
Hamachek, D.E., 63, 64, 78, 79, 88, 89, 90, 96, 111, 113, 121, 123, 133, 134, 145, 203, 214, 231, 264
Handicap, 13-14
Harley, R.K., 55
Harshberger, C., 218
Hartman, D., 41, 42, 68, 69, 81, 89, 133, 134, 162, 172, 209, 245
Hatlen, P., 52
Head, C., 56, 57, 151
Henderson, L.T., 41, 49, 130, 163, 169, 214, 271, 281
Hickford, J., 25, 72, 77
Hicks, S., 155, 157, 171, 186, 188, 224, 231
Historical perspective, 8-12
Hocken, S., 7, 16, 22, 26, 42, 97, 102, 161, 162, 169, 235, 271, 282
Hope, 153, 199-201
Horney, K., 64, 115, 123, 128, 137, 229
Hostility, 177-178, 182, 220, 266
Humor, role of, 44, 241, 242

I

Identity, 196-197
Independence (*see* Dependence)
Intelligence, 52-53, 244
Interpersonal relationships, 38, 77, 82-88, 186, 229-231, 268, 269, 288
Irwin, R., 29
Isolation, 40, 153, 154, 177-178, 182

J

James, W., 62, 79, 102, 107, 109, 111, 115
Jan, J., 245, 255
Jervis, F.M., 55, 56, 151
Jones, W.P., 210
Jourard, S.M., 64, 67, 70, 137, 186, 207, 214

K

Kappan, D., 23
Keegan, D.L., 240
Kelley, J., 37
Kemper, R.G., 6, 53, 87, 115, 124, 172, 177, 183, 190, 205, 212, 223, 249, 254, 284
Kirchner, C., 17, 33
Kirtley, D.D., 14, 18, 19, 38, 45, 149
Klein, G.S., 52

Klich, B., 196
Krents, H., 14, 42, 43, 44, 70, 75, 80, 81, 87, 108, 165, 176, 199, 255, 259, 271
Kübler-Ross, E., 154

L

LaBenne, W.L., 64, 68, 96, 104, 108, 111, 127, 145, 211, 280, 284
Lambert, R.M., 149, 188, 207, 214
Land, S.L., 265
Lazarus, R.S., 206
Ledwith, B.E., 56
Legally blind, definition, 12
Locke, D., 289
Losses, 184-186, 191, 199
Lowenfeld, B., 8, 10, 11, 19, 33, 35, 37, 38, 45, 52, 55, 66, 245, 266, 279
Low vision, 13, 20, 27, 247
    (*see also* Visual loss)
Lukoff, I., 45, 97, 149
Lunt, L., 28, 51, 134, 232, 270

M

Maladaptive behavior, 171, 177-178, 188-189, 196, 213-216, 222
Mangold, S.S., 96, 103, 108, 201, 221, 289
Maslow, A.H., 64, 65, 115, 117, 137
Mayadas, N.S., 96
McAndrew, H., 95, 108
McCandless, B.R., 125, 126, 284
McCoy, M.B., 36, 135, 166, 175, 180, 187, 193, 224, 269
Mead, G.H., 64, 79, 115
Mehta, V., 28, 86, 245, 260, 272
Meighan, T., 56, 57, 151
Meyerson, L., 45, 81
Miller, W.H., 149, 151, 192
Mitchell, M., 31, 43, 51, 76, 161, 168, 174, 178, 185, 243, 260, 274
Mobilization, 153, 205, 209
Models, 43-44, 70, 218, 260-261
Monbeck, M.E., 45
Moore, V.B., 24, 34, 46, 226, 241, 266
Moos, R.H., 122, 156, 210, 239, 244, 255
Morgan, B.K., 83, 165
Mourning, 153, 175-181, 253
Multihandicapped, 250-252
Murphree, O.D., 149
Mussen, P.H., 241

N

Napier, G., 50
National Society to Prevent Blindness, 16, 17
Needham, W.E., 252
Neu, C., 239, 255
Newman, D.K., 241
Norris, M., 19

O

Oehler-Giarratana, J., 249
Ohnstad, K., 40, 261
Ophthalmologist (*see* Physician)
Orientation and mobility, 22-29
    cane, 24
    dog guide, 25-26
    electronic travel aids, 26-27
    sighted guide, 23-24

P

Palomares, U., 289
Parad, H.J., 210
Parent (*see* Significant other)
Parkes, C.M., 171
Partially seeing, definition, 12
Passing, 132
Passivity, 41
Personal attributes (PA) (*see* Attributes, personal)
Personality traits, 53, 155, 239-242
Peterson, R., 17, 33
Physician, 154, 167-169, 253-255
Pierce, R., 212
Potok, A., 15, 39, 101, 177, 194, 223, 224
Professional role, 167-169, 173-175, 179-181, 189-193, 201-205, 216-223, 233-236, 280-284, 284-296
Psychological consequences of blindness, 49-57
Psychology of blindness (*see* Blindness, psychology of)
Putnam, P., 129, 195, 244

R

Rapp, D.W., 116, 279
Reaffirmation, 193-205
Reassessment, 193-205
Recreation, 35-37
Referent group, 80, 102

Rejection of aids, 27, 32, 155
Resnick, R., 12, 164, 246
Resources, 209, 254, 259-260
Richard, C., 36, 252
Riffenburgh, R., 154, 179, 213, 214
Ritz, D., 96, 265
Roberts, A., 22, 212, 264
Rogers, C., 64, 91, 115, 122, 126, 128, 137, 201, 227, 229, 268
Role models (*see* Models)
Role playing, 219, 291-294
Rosenberg, M., 137
Routh, T., 147, 149, 192, 205, 210, 218, 230, 231
Rusalem, H., 33, 34, 221, 240, 259, 261
Russell, R., 33, 86, 124, 166, 186, 227

S

Safilio-Rothschild, C., 248
Sams, T.A., 67
Schindele, R., 151
Scholl, G.T., 33, 49, 67
Schulz, P., 38, 41, 54, 146, 172, 173, 175, 177, 178, 186, 188, 189, 191, 200, 207, 214, 225, 241, 242, 249, 253, 254, 255, 257
Scott, E.P., 245, 255
Scott, R.A., 43, 61
Secord, P.F., 67
Self, 76, 115, 123-126, 160, 197, 267
    definition, 62
Self-acceptance, 150, 152, 196, 206, 218, 223-236, 261, 279, 284-287
Self-concept, 47, 56-57, 145, 153, 160
    definition, 63
    development of, 66-68
Self-consciousness, 39, 213, 221
Self-esteem, 12, 56-57, 107, 119-120, 145, 152, 222, 223-236, 261, 262, 265, 279-280, 284-287, 287-296
    competence model, 91-120
        summary diagram, 119
    definition, 6, 63, 228
    development of, 5, 61-90, 110, 118, 222
    external sources of, 61-90
    high self-esteem, 95, 137-140, 228
    impact of visual loss on, 6, 22, 29, 32, 35, 37, 47-49, 81
    increased self-esteem, 155, 199, 208, 213, 218, 259
    internal sources of, 91-120
    lowered self-esteem, 164, 176, 183, 184, 275
    low self-esteem, 137, 140-141, 153, 242
    measurement of, 65
    reflective model, 61, 68-70, 76
Self-evaluation, 88-90, 101-105
Self-pity, 154, 175, 178, 182, 212
Self-presentation, 73
Self-rejection, 104, 164, 225, 231
Severson, A.L., 146,149
Shaffer, L.F., 121
Sheppard, W., 35, 189, 215, 261
Shoben, E.J., 121
Shock, 153, 155, 170-174, 250
Significant others (SO), 68-70, 79-82, 89, 91-120, 160, 162, 189, 220, 253, 260, 263, 271, 280
    adjusting process, 255-259
Simpkins, K., 52
Sloan, S., 254
Smithdas, R.J., 251, 252
Social relationships (*see* Interpersonal relationships)
Sociological consequences of blindness, 38-49
Sommers, V., 38, 56, 149, 151, 257
Spaulding, P.J., 19
Sperber, A., 7, 15, 73, 98, 131, 160, 186, 196, 216, 223, 253, 254, 261
Spouse (*see* Significant others)
Spread, 72, 197
Standards, 101-106
Steinzor, L.V., 229
Stephens, W.B., 52
Stevens, J.O., 289
Stogner, P.C., 250
Stotland, E., 99
Stringer, L.A., 63, 64, 91, 137, 212
Success, 107-111
Succumbing, 84, 181-193
Sullivan, H.S., 66, 76, 89, 122
Sullivan, T., 41, 68, 85, 178, 183, 228, 273
Support network, 209, 234, 253
    (*see also* Significant others)
Suterko, S., 21
Swallow, R., 53
Symonds, P.M., 89, 107

T

Thume, L., 149
Thurber, J., 101, 173
Trauma, 160-169, 255, 263
    definition, 160
    onset of visual loss, 160-162, 170,
        253, 262
    preparation for, 161, 253
    social, 162-165, 169, 176
    subsequent, 165-167
Trismen, D.A., 52
Tsu, V.B., 122, 156, 210, 239, 244, 255
Tuttle, D.W., 21, 29, 30

U

Ulrich, S., 258, 260
Underberg, R.P., 56, 149, 151, 247, 257

V

Vajda, A., 185, 232, 272
Values, 111-115, 194, 197-199, 252-253
VanderKolk, C.J., 34, 52, 172, 186, 200,
    221, 240, 241
Verbalism, 51
Verrillo, R.T., 56, 149, 151, 247, 257
Vineberg, S.E., 265
Visibility of disability, 15, 248
Visual loss
    degree of, 20, 247-249
    stability of, 249-250
Visually disabled, 14

Visually handicapped, 13-14
Visually impaired (VI), 13, 68-70

W

Weinberg, J.R., 67
Wells, H., 280, 284, 289
Welsh, R., 25, 29, 100, 110, 192, 204,
    218, 268
Wenkart, A., 62
West, M., 149, 188, 207, 214
Whiteman, M., 97, 149
Wierig, G.J., 196
Wilson, M.E., 48
Withdrawal, 41, 153, 154, 175, 177-178,
    182, 194
Wright, B.A., 14, 45, 48, 53, 55, 70, 72,
    88, 127, 128, 131, 137, 148, 175, 178,
    182, 183, 195, 198, 203, 206, 211, 216,
    225, 233, 249
Wyder, F.T., 48
Wylie, R., 228, 229

Y

Yank, B., 217
Yates, E., 234, 244, 257
Yoder, N., 82
Younie, W., 221

Z

Zunich, M., 56